Progress
in
Toxicology

Special Topics

Volume 1

Progress
in
Toxicology

Special Topics

Volume 1

Gerhard Zbinden

SPRINGER-VERLAG NEW YORK · HEIDELBERG · BERLIN

GERHARD ZBINDEN, M.D.
Laboratory of Experimental and Toxicological Pathology
Institute of Pathological Anatomy
University of Zurich
Zurich, Switzerland

Library of Congress Cataloging in Publication Data

Zbinden, Gerhard, 1924
Progress in toxicology.

1. Drugs—Toxicology.   I. Title.
RA1238.Z34   615.9   73-12957

© 1973 by Springer-Verlag New York Inc.

Printed in the United States of America.

ISBN 0-387-06495-8   Springer-Verlag New York · Heidelberg · Berlin
ISBN 3-540-06495-8   Springer-Verlag Berlin · Heidelberg · New York

Contents

I.	**Introduction**	**1**
	Special Topics	1
	The Many Faces of Toxicology	2
II.	**Formal Toxicology**	**4**
	Toxicological Prerequisites for the Study and General Release of New Drugs	4
	Towards a Comprehensive and Methodical Approach to Toxicology	17
	Acute Toxicology	23
III.	**Speculative Toxicology**	**28**
	General Remarks	28
	Induction of Drug Metabolizing Enzymes	28
	Protein Binding	33
	Pyridoxal Phosphate	36
IV.	**Comparative Toxicology**	**38**
	General Remarks	38
	The Factor Age	38
	Ambient Temperature	43
V.	**Pharmacodynamic Toxicology**	**46**
	General Remarks	46
	Thyroid Stimulation	46
VI.	**Symptomatic Toxicology**	**49**
	General Remarks	49
	Oxaluria	49
	Acute, Interstitial, Eosinophilic Myocarditis	52
	Coombs Test Positivity	54
VII.	**Systematic Toxicology**	**56**
	General Remarks	56
	Hexachlorophene	56
	Hypervitaminosis	60
VIII.	**Geographical Toxicology**	**66**
	General Remarks	66
	Subacute, Myelo-optico Neuropathy	67
	Index	**86**

I

INTRODUCTION

SPECIAL TOPICS

I was then Director of Biological Research of a pharmaceutical
company just west of the Hackensack River swamps when my collaborators presented me with an impressive book. Its gold-embossed title
read: "WHAT I KNOW ABOUT BIOLOGICAL RESEARCH by GERHARD ZBINDEN,
M.D.". Those acquainted with the subtleties of American humor will
have guessed the book's content: about 700 empty pages. But I liked
the idea enough to write down what I knew about my branch of biological research, drug toxicology. With gentle prodding by Dr. Parkhurst
Shore of Dallas, Texas, I assembled a review on those experimental
and clinical aspects of drug toxicology with which I, as an industrial
toxicologist, had been most concerned with. It turned out to be a
modest paper, considerably less than 700 pages, but it seemed to fill
a need for others who were laboring on similar problems (Zbinden 1963).

Drug toxicology has changed much since 1963 when the review appeared. Its problems have certainly not become smaller. Scientists
of many biological specialties have become interested in questions of
harmful drug effects. Their input has greatly enriched the knowledge
of the basic processes underlying certain forms of toxic drug reactions. With this surge of interest and effort, extreme specialization
has occurred which sometimes tended to dominate the toxicological
scene. Stimulation of drug metabolizing enzymes, for example, is
analyzed to the finest details of enzyme kinetics and ultrastructural
adaptation, but its significance as a cause or modulator of drug
toxicity is still poorly understood. Genetic damage, dramatically
demonstrated in elegant experimental systems, is another interesting
field where specialization spreads rapidly and where it becomes most
difficult to understand the meaning of the intricate tests for the
day-to-day use of drugs. It seemed appropriate, therefore, to update
my 10 year old paper.

It would have been attractive to team up with colleagues and
write a textbook of drug toxicology. But the field has become so
broad and is developing so fast that too much time would have to be
spent to cover all fronts. It was my editor, Prof. Angermeier, who
suggested that I might do better to deal with just a few aspects of
toxicology at one time and to issue short essays at frequent intervals. This is how "Special Topics" have come into existence.

In these booklets I intend to present, in a not too solemn way,
what I have learned about toxic effects of drugs in animals and man.

It is what my teachers, friends, and collaborators have taught me,
what I have selected from the immense scientific literature, and what
I have seen in my laboratory. Thus, most of it is neither my own
work nor necessarily based on my own ideas. I only claim credit for
interpretations and extrapolations. They are one man's opinion, and
because of that, bound to be subjective and, as time goes on, liable
to change.

I cannot thank all those who over the years have shared their
knowledge and ideas with me and whose work I am utilizing freely. To
select one for all, I want to express my gratitude to my friend and
teacher, Professor Alfred Studer, of Basel, Switzerland, whose scientific ideas and results are an integral part of these Special Topics.

THE MANY FACES OF TOXICOLOGY

There are still people who believe with Webster's Dictionary
that toxicology is nothing but the science of poisons. For them, a
toxicologist is a man whom one can call at any hour when the baby has
licked mother's facial cream and the cat has eaten a poisoned mouse.
True enough, one important part of toxicology is indeed concerned with
acute intoxications. But those readers who have bought this booklet
to learn about poisoning and antidotes should bring it back to the
bookstore immediately because this particular branch of toxicology
will barely be discussed. Those who have purchased it to read about
air pollution, dangerous pesticides, and harmful food additives have
also made a bad investment, and so have those who would like to use
the science of poisons to exterminate whatever living creature is
molesting them.

This booklet is about undesired effects of drugs which, by all
accounts, have become one of the important causes of disease. But if
you think that the major effort in toxicology today is to explain and
perhaps treat those undesired effects, you are mistaken. Most of the
working hours of the practicing toxicologist are filled with demon-
strating safety, i.e., lack of toxicity. He does this in a certain
way predetermined by tradition and official regulations. This is the
realm of FORMAL TOXICOLOGY, an activity which has become a multi-
million dollar enterprise. It produces the safety data on which
clinical trials and marketing of new drugs depend. Since it too has
become very specialized, some aspects of formal toxicology and the
directions in which it seems to develop will be discussed in the subsequent chapter.

It is sometimes said that one can tell a toxicologist by his
worried look. This is understandable in view of the fact that his
standard procedures often do not disclose any specific toxic action
of a new drug. With such an experiment the toxicologist has done all
he can to establish the new drug's safety, knowing only too well that
there probably is no such thing as a safe or non-toxic drug. To deal
with this difficult situation, he has created what one might call
SPECULATIVE TOXICOLOGY. This is a most interesting approach which
tries to anticipate harmful effects from sources other than the
toxicological experiment, e.g., the chemical and physical properties
of the compounds, their pharmacokinetic behavior, their influence on
enzymatic processes; in short, from any quality a careful chemical
and biological evaluation can uncover.

It is, of course, also possible that the toxicological tests will disclose a harmful effect of a new drug. As a matter of fact, toxicological experiments are so designed that this is most likely to happen. The problem to worry about in this instance is the decision whether or not the observed injury is of significance for the use of the drug in man. In such a situation one must first investigate whether the animal system which signaled the toxic effect is likely to be representative for man. This is the subject matter of COMPARATIVE TOXICOLOGY. If the test system is considered relevant, the concepts of PHARMACODYNAMIC TOXICOLOGY must be applied. They help to decide whether or not the conditions under which the toxicity developed in the experimental animal would be similar when the drug is used therapeutically in patients.

Three more branches of toxicology shall be briefly mentioned. One might be called SYMPTOMATIC TOXICOLOGY. It is popular with clinicians who like to study a symptom or a syndrome or, best of all, a full-blown disease. The goal is to identify the offending drug and to unravel the mechanism by which it has caused the so-called disease of medical progress. To do this one must often have recourse to animal experiments; thus comparative, pharmacodynamic, and speculative toxicology may all be needed to solve the problems. Secondly, there is SYSTEMATIC TOXICOLOGY. It starts out with the chemical substances which are classified according to structure, physical properties, or pharmacological activities. Toxicological data are collected and listed together with the other qualities. This documentation is useful to the clinician as background information and should ultimately lead to a better understanding of structure-activity relationships in toxicology. Lastly, GEOGRAPHICAL TOXICOLOGY shall be mentioned. It is concerned with the puzzling phenomenon that certain toxic drug reactions seem to be more frequent in particular countries or on one continent. It analyzes various factors which might account for these differences, e.g., climate, nutritional practices, racial influences, prescribing habits, infectious diseases, and other environmental influences.

II

FORMAL TOXICOLOGY

TOXICOLOGICAL PREREQUISITES FOR THE STUDY
AND GENERAL RELEASE OF NEW DRUGS

The Rules of the Game

Any new drug must be submitted to a set of animal tests before it may be given to man. Moreover, an additional series of experiments must be completed prior to its release for commercial distribution. The current experimental procedures have been described by innumerable reviewers and expert committees. And true to the elementary law of advertising that the message will be believed if it is repeated time and again, toxicologists and governmental regulatory agencies have almost universally accepted a well-defined experimental approach to safety testing of new drugs.

To the uninitiated a conventional toxicological work-up of a new drug looks like a curious collection of data notable by its super-abundance of extravagantly accurate test results on the one hand, and by the lack of desirable pieces of information on the other. For a new topical preparation for example, it may give the precise median lethal doses of the active ingredient in rats and mice and perhaps a third species after both oral and parenteral application including the 95% confidence limits and a detailed list of symptoms preceding death. But it must not, and often does not, contain any information about the drug's penetration through inflamed skin. The data sheet of a new tranquilizer may list the results of over 2,000 liver function tests obtained in scores of rats, dogs, and monkeys (usually remaining within normal range) but is often silent about the new drug's ability to potentiate alcohol and general anesthetics and its effect on ethanol metabolism.

Critics and skeptics are assured that the toxicological proce-dures are meant to remain flexible and that the rules for safety testing of new drugs are merely guidelines which must not be followed to the letter. This statement is not true. There are already several toxicological procedures issued in writing by governmental regulatory agencies which must be performed as directed. There will be more of these in the future. Moreover, toxicologists fear -- not without reason -- that any significant deviation from the generally accepted guidelines may be questioned by reviewers at regulatory agencies. And while there are numerous enlightened government officials who are responsive to a rational approach to safety testing, chances are that the data may also be judged by others who insist on a strict observance of their favorite set of guidelines. As a consequence and in order to avoid any delay, the guideline which will satisfy the most demanding health authority becomes the generally accepted procedure. A look at the preclinical data sheets of new drugs regardless of their origin readily discloses that standardization of toxicological procedures has become an undeniable fact. Differences still exist with regard to certain experimental details, such as the number of animals and the duration of treatment. But since drugs are often developed to be distributed throughout the entire world, the most comprehensive and thus the generally acceptable version of the test procedure is usually performed.

Guidelines and standard procedures are not without merits. Above all, they assure that a comprehensive set of toxicological data is gathered with each new drug before it is given to humans. They facilitate comparison with related and clinically proven drugs, and they serve as a convenient alibi should anything go wrong later. Standardization of toxicological procedures also make it possible to amass the bulk of experimental data with the help of automated procedures and with personnel of limited technical skill. Best of all, the usefulness and relevance of standard procedures can be evaluated by direct observation in man, thus providing impetus and scientific background for improvements. This is a difficult task of great importance which makes toxicology one of the most attractive and relevant fields of applied biology.

Toxicological Test Procedures

When the pioneers of toxicology decided that harmful effects of new drugs should be assessed in animals rather than through heroic self-administration, two principal experimental approaches had to be considered. One was the pharmacological approach which required a specially designed experiment for each toxicological effect. Since there were numerous harmful drug reactions already known and many more that could be imagined, the attempt to develop such a large number of standardized assay methods looked like a futile endeavour. The obvious solution seemed to lie with a medical approach. Consequently, an omnibus procedure evolved in which animals were forced to take the drug just as patients would at a later stage. A battery of clinical and laboratory methods were employed to catch any harmful effect as it occurred. To improve the probability of recognizing as many undesired effects as possible, the toxicological tests deviated from the clinical situation in four ways: 1) Drugs were given at higher than the therapeutic dose, 2) animals got them for very long periods of time, 3) routes of administration not expected to be used in man were admissible, and 4) the treated subjects were killed at the end of the study to permit autopsy and histopathology of the organs.

Two types of experiments were selected, namely the acute toxicity test in which drugs were given once or a few times at the most, and subacute or chronic tests where treatment was continued over a certain period of time. The acute toxicity experiment was conceived to give an all or none answer -- death or no death -- over a broad range of dose levels from which the median lethal dose could be calculated.

TABLE 1

Prolonged Toxicity Studies

Subject	Generally Accepted Procedure	Major Alternatives Still Under Discussion
Animal Species	1 rodent (rat), 1 nonrodent (dog), third species if significant toxicity occurs.	Always third species. Monkey, pig, mouse, rabbit, cat or which? Species which metabolize drug or which respond pharmacologically like man. Inbred or random-bred, conventional or specified pathogen free animals. Litter mates equally divided among groups. One or more defined strains.
Feeding	ad libitum	Paired feeding of treated and controls.
Number of Test Groups	At least 3 and 1 control.	or more.
Magnitude of Doses	Highest: must cause significant toxicity; lowest: small multiple of therapeutic dose in mg/kg. Others in between.	Adjustment of dose depending on age, general tolerance, etc. Determination of dose depending on blood or tissue levels. Special procedures for poorly absorbed, pharmacologically highly active, cytotoxic (irritant) or extremely non-toxic drugs.
Number of Animals per Group	Rodents: at least 10 of each sex; nonrodent: at least 5 of each sex.	Larger groups. Groups large enough to permit meaningful statistical treatment.
Duration of Treatment	2 weeks to several years depending on projected human use (see Table 2).	---
Routes and Frequency of Administration	Same routes as projected for use in man. Oral: admixture to diet or 6x intubation per week. Parenteral: 6x weekly.	Routes which assure maximal blood or tissue level, frequency of administration which assures continuous levels or levels similar to those obtained in clinical use in man. Interrupted administration to minimize adaptation. Daily treatment. Treatment schedule as in clinical use.
Age of Animals	Rats: start with immature animals. Dogs: 1 year.	Studies on newborn and very old animals.
Reversibility	Not part of routine procedure.	Special groups treated and taken off drugs after various time periods and for various lengths of time.
Measurements and Observations	Weight, appearance, eye examination.	Food and water consumption, food efficiency, reflexes, behavioral tests, ECG, EEG, neuromuscular and psychomotor function, sexual behavior, memory, etc.

Hematology	Before test, after 1,2,3,6, 9,12,etc. months in part of test animals. RBC, hematocrit, Hb, WBC, diff. count, platelet count, reticulocyte count, prothrombin time.	Examine all animals. ESR, red cell fragility, metHb, other coagulation tests, bone marrow examination, spleen and lymph node cytology, phagocytic activity, etc.
Blood Chemistry	In nonrodent: SGPT, alk. phosphatase, BUN, serum creatinine, fasting blood sugar, plasma proteins, bilirubin.	Selected or all animals including rodents. Additional enzyme and organ function tests, electrolytes, clearance studies, cholesterol, total lipids, triglycerides.
Urinalysis	Nonrodent: spec. gravity, sugar, protein, bile, ketone, pH, sediment.	Selected or all animals including rodents. Total volume, electrolytes, enzymes.
Autopsy	Complete, in part of rodents and all nonrodents. Weight of liver, kidney, testicle, ovary.	Complete, in all animals. Weight of additional organs, e.g., thyroid, adrenals, uterus, epididymis, heart, etc.
Histopathology	15-20 major organs, routine staining.	More organs and tissues, special staining methods, histochemistry, electron microscopy.
Known Standard Drug	Not part of routine procedure.	Treatment of one or more groups with known standard drug (positive control).

Special Studies

Reproduction- Teratology	Fertility and reproduction study in rats. Teratological study in rabbits and mice or rats. Perinatal and postnatal study in rats.	Use of various strains, e.g., with propensity to develop certain type of malformation. Use of primates.
Mutagenicity	Not part of routine procedure (yet).	In selected cases or with all drugs? In vitro cytogenetics with human, animal, or plant cells. In vivo cytogenetics. Host mediated assays with different indicator organisms. Dominant lethal test. Specific locus test. High dose, therapeutic dose, acute, subacute or chronic treatment?
Carcinogenicity	Not part of routine procedure (yet).	In selected cases or with all drugs? Long term studies in rodents. One or more species, one or more strains? Use of dogs, non-human primates. Short term screening tests.
Drug Interactions	Combined LD_{50} with drugs likely to be used in combination with new drug.	Combined subacute and chronic tests. Potentiation or inhibition of specific pharmacological and toxicological effects.

This procedure has not materially changed over the years. Some additional clinical observations are now customarily gathered, but little or no laboratory examinations are done. More about this important experiment and about the conclusions toxicologists and clinicians may draw from it is found on pages 23-27.

The creative energies and the fire of perfectionism of toxicologists have chiefly been aimed at the prolonged toxicity studies. These tests used to be called "subacute" if they were of short duration, perhaps up to 3 months, and "chronic" if they lasted longer. There are no other differences. The main reason why short term, subacute experiments are done is to permit initiation of studies in man, whereas chronic toxicity tests are deemed necessary for broad clinical trials and for marketing.

The basic procedures for prolonged toxicity studies are essentially determined by tradition and continuously reconfirmed by expert committees of the scientific, industrial, and regulatory establishment. They differ only with regard to the extent to which the individual toxicologist is willing to push his perfectionism. The generally accepted procedures can be summarized in a few sentences (Table 1). But we must remember that many experimental details are far from being settled. In the table they are listed as Major Alternatives.

When To Do What

What should be known about a new drug before it is given for the first time to a human being? How much toxicological testing should be done prior to initiation of limited and extended clinical trials? How much is needed to grant permission for marketing? These questions are hotly debated by clinical pharmacologists who bear the burden of responsibility for the safe conduct of clinical trials but sometimes feel unduly hampered in their work by having to wait for the completion of routine animal experiments. The answer, of course, depends on the pharmacological, pharmacokinetic, and chemical properties of the compound, its metabolism, affinities to tissues, and mechanism of action. In other words, what should be known is not easy to come by. What must be available on paper, however, can be stated in a few words: Guidelines issued by experts and adhered to rigidly by regulatory agencies provide the ready answer. The nature of the toxicological information required is identical all over the world, but there are many differences with regard to the extent of testing considered adequate in various countries. Hebold (1972) has collected current recommendations of several official and semiofficial bodies. With his permission his summary table is reproduced (Table 2).

Looking at this table, is it not surprising that the amount of toxicological information deemed necessary to permit clinical trials depends exclusively on the length of time the drug will be taken by the patients? This concept was perhaps not invented but strongly supported by the former FDA chief pharmacologist, A.J. Lehman. He mentioned it first in a short paper published in 1959 and perfected it in a much renowned talk in 1963. Mimeographed copies of his slides were circulated widely among toxicologists and soon reached the status

TABLE 2

SYNOPSIS OF DURATION OF TOXICOLOGY STUDIES FOR ANIMALS IN DIFFERENT COUNTRIES
(from Hebold 1972)

Duration of human administration	USA	Gr. Brit.	FRG	Sweden	Switz.
single dose		21 days	2-4 weeks	2-4 weeks	not less than 14 days
several days up to 1 week	2 weeks	39 days		3 months	
up to 2 weeks	2 weeks- 3 months				not more than 3 months required
up to 1 month		90 days			
over 1 month		180 days	3-6 months		
up to 3 months	4 weeks- 6 months				
6 months to unlimited	3 months- 12 months dogs 18 months rats				

	USSR	EEC	WHO	ESSDT*
single dose		2-4 weeks	less than 3 months	1-3 weeks
several days up to 1 week	10 days			1 month
up to 2 weeks	30 days			3 months
up to 1 month	2-6 months		3-6 months	
over 1 month		3-6 months		
up to 3 months				
6 months to unlimited				

* European Society for the Study of Drug Toxicity

of secret guidelines. Although the concept was later amended and extended, the basic philosophy remained unchanged.

It appears reasonable, though, to include considerations other than the length of the proposed treatment in man when toxicological prerequisites for new drugs are discussed. The major factor which should determine the amount of preclinical testing is, of course, the drug's own toxic potential. Since this is at least partly related to its pharmacological properties, the experienced investigator should be able to make a preliminary determination of the nature and severity of the toxic effects from the results of the pharmacological evaluation and plan the toxicological tests accordingly. Moreover, it is possible to design an open-ended toxicological test which delivers information continuously and does not last for a predetermined time period. With such a procedure the decisions to start clinical trials, to extend or to continue them with higher doses can be made any time.

TABLE 3

A Simplified Example of a Discretionary Toxicity Study in Rats

Group	Dose mg/kg	Observations	Days of Treatment					
			2	4	8	16	32	64
			Number of Animals with Symptom or Organ Change					
I	x	no change	10	10	10	10	10	10
II	5 x	Lymphopenia	0	1	0	0	0	0
		Thymus atrophy	2	2	0	0	0	0
		Retard.growth	6	5	8	3	1	1
III	25 x	Retard.growth	10	10	10	10	10	10
		Lymphopenia	2	10	8	0	0	0
		Thymus atrophy	4	6	3	1	3	1
		Inhib.sperm maturat.	0	0	0	0	2	3
		Gastric ulcer	0	2	10	0	0	0
		Fatty change liver	0	0	1	0	2	1
Contr	0	Inhib.sperm maturat.	0	0	0	0	0	0
		Fatty change liver	0	0	0	0	1	2
Clinical Trials			hold	hold	hold	single dose absorpt.study	mult. dose toler.	double blind efficacy
Additional Animal Tests (based on observations during toxicity studies)			none	gastric secretion ulcus production in other species effect of atropin	none		dominant lethal test	effect on spermato-genesis
Clinical Observation			--	--	--	long T 1/2	well toler.	very ef-fective
Additional Studies (based on clinical observations)						Clearance biliary excret. protein binding	none	none

To do this toxicity test, one starts with a relatively large number of animals. They are observed for about one week and then treatment with 3 dose levels is started. Groups of treated and control animals are sacrificed at logarithmically spaced points in time or at other convenient time intervals. Hematological and biochemical tests are done before sacrifice and histology of the major organs is performed promptly. Adjustment of dose upwards or downwards is possible. If no serious toxicity is detected, the first clinical trials, e.g., single dose absorption studies, may be started after 2 to 4 weeks. As time passes, additional toxicological information pours in. Based on this continuously updated documentation, clinical studies can either be extended gradually, held at the same level or reduced. Conversely, early clinical observations can point to some unexpected and undesired effect and in turn give reason for modifying or amplifying the animal experiment. I have once called this concept the ping-pong approach to preclinical toxicity testing. This is not a particularly original name (discretionary toxicity test might be better), but it indicates that an interplay of two partners -- the toxicologist and the clinical pharmacologist -- is needed to expedite the development of a new drug. A simplified and hypothetical example is shown in Table 4.

Pragmatic toxicologists will find many deficiencies with this method. They will criticize the small number of animals sacrificed at any one time, the sin of omission not to conduct hematological and chemical tests before starting the experiment and many other deviations from the lawful path. They will have to admit, though, that the approach provides rapid information about early drug effects which are often missed if one autopsies animals only after several weeks or months of treatment. They will also have to acknowledge the usefulness of the built-in steering mechanism which permits monitoring and special consideration of observed or suspected toxic reactions and provides information about reversibility of functional and morphological changes. Furthermore, the detailed examination of groups of animals at logarithmically spaced intervals permits establishment of dose-effect and time-effect curves even for morphological changes. Such curves are often useful particularly for the evaluation of irreversible and cumulative toxicity. Finally, the ping-pong method of toxicity testing also enables one to stop the game should signs of serious toxicity develop in the animal experiment. Efforts may be shifted to other projects and time is saved -- time, one of the few things money does not buy.

A similar method was developed by toxicologists of the National Cancer Institute (1969). It provides intensive exposure of relatively few animals followed by elaborate clinical-pharmacological and pharmacokinetic studies. A summary of the procedure is shown in Table 4. It is particularly useful for anticancer drugs whose toxic effects are at least partly predictable and can usually be detected early by clinical and laboratory methods.

Each route of administration requires its own toxicological evaluation. Never can the method of administration of a drug to man be changed without a consideration of the toxicological consequences. Animal testing is usually necessary, but it may often be sufficient to assess only the pharmacokinetic consequences of the changed route of administration. For the topical use of drugs simple but useful tests methods exist. They measure local tolerance and general

TABLE 4

General Protocol for Preclinical Toxicology of the Laboratory
of Toxicology, National Cancer Institute (1969)

Type I Toxicology

Study 1   Acute and Chronic Lethality in Mice

Oral and parenteral application of drug, single and five day treatment

Study 2   Single Dose Toxicity in Beagle Dogs

Parenteral or oral dosing of single animals to reach toxic level.
Extensive clinical and laboratory studies over a 45 day (or longer)
period, autopsy and histopathology

Study 3   24 Hour Intravenous Infusion in Beagle Dogs

Clinical and laboratory studies and autopsy as in Study 2

Study 4   Five Day Daily Dosing in Beagle Dogs

Drug administration to groups of 2 dogs. Additional groups are added
if signs of toxicity are not reached.
At end of treatment 1 dog sacrificed, 1 dog observed as in Study 2.
2 additional dogs treated with dose that caused mild toxicity on a
5 day on, 9 day off, 5 day on course, then observed for 30 days.
Clinical observation, laboratory tests and pathology as in Study 2.

Type II Toxicology   To gain further information on predictability and reversibility of toxic effects discovered in Type I Toxicology.

Procedures Studies in dogs and primates specifically designed to reflect proposed
clinical use, pharmacokinetic behavior and pharmacodynamic properties.

Type III Toxicology To define the toxicity of drug alone or in combination prior
to large scale, long term clinical trials.

Procedures Specially designed according to the results of early clinical trials.
Dosage schedule and duration of treatment planned considering pharmacokinetic behavior and pharmacologic effects. Number of animals and
duration of treatment is gradually increased.

toxicity. They should always be performed. Particular care should
be taken when a drug is administered by inhalation. Absorption may
be very rapid and detoxification can differ considerably from that
occurring after oral or i.v. application. Extensive acute and chronic studies on small and large animals including metabolism must therefore precede any use of the compounds in man.

The Problem of Teratogenic, Carcinogenic and Mutagenic Hazards

Clinical pharmacologists are convinced that early evaluation of
new drugs in man can safely be conducted in specialized research units
where patients are monitored around the clock by experienced physicians
and a trained nursing staff. But even under the most favorable conditions, certain forms of drug toxicity, i.e., the slowly developing,
cumulative and irreversible organ damage, can often not be recognized.
Teratogenic, carcinogenic and mutagenic effects are the most ominous
of these irreversible injuries. Guiding principles must therefore be

adopted which will reduce these hazards to an absolute minimum.

To avoid teratogenic damage, pregnant women must be excluded from all early drug trials. The responsibility that this precaution is observed rests with the clinical investigator. It is sometimes suggested that all females of childbearing age should be excluded from such trials because they often do not know that they have become pregnant. I submit that they usually do know, and if instructed properly, will inform, perhaps not the clinical investigator, but certainly the nurse or another female on the staff.

As clinical studies are extended, a close contact with the patients is no longer possible. At this time the teratogenic potential of the new drug should be known from animal experiments. A negative outcome of such studies, of course, does not preclude that the compound may still be teratogenic in man. But there are hardly any other realistic options open, and one can never arrive at an absolute certitude. Only through extensive clinical experience will the lingering doubts ultimately be dispelled.

The carcinogenic and mutagenic hazards of new drugs are even more difficult to avoid. Except for a few classes of drugs, we lack the essential knowledge to predict these effects accurately or even to comprehend the magnitude of the risk. Animal experiments are available with which strong carcinogens and mutagens can be identified. Many of these agents belong to the group of anticancer and immuno-suppressant drugs. There is no need to conduct lengthy carcinogenic-ity and mutagenicity tests with such drugs before starting clinical trials, since these compounds would not be tested in man unless their therapeutic potential was considered very important, so much so that a positive outcome of the tests would not alter the decision. After such a drug has shown promising therapeutic results, the carcinogenic and mutagenic potential should be evaluated in animal tests so that the full spectrum of its biological action will be known. And only after the completion and careful evaluation of the test results can the question of extending clinical trials to diseases other than malignancies be discussed.

The situation becomes even less transparent when we consider weak carcinogens and weak mutagens. Any chemical substance whose lack of carcinogenic and mutagenic effect has not been proven with certainty should be considered a weak carcinogen or mutagen. When tested with the presently available in vitro and in vivo methods, their carcinogenic and mutagenic properties are either so weak that positive effects have not yet been discovered, or they are such that a hint of positive action is only seen under special circumstances, e.g., when tests are done with extremely high doses or concentrations, in selected species or strains of animals or with unphysiological in vitro systems. With this facetious definition I want to make clear that a large number of chemicals in our environment, including old and new drugs, might be weak carcinogens and mutagens. Thus, the question when to test new drugs for carcinogenic and mutagenic effects represents only a tiny element of a much larger problem.

For the future of drug research, the tiny element may become a fateful issue. Mutagenic and carcinogenic tests as presently performed are time consuming. To require completion of these tests before permitting clinical trials to start, would markedly slow down

the flow of new drugs. Moreover, the routine animal tests as present
ly performed, are not satisfactory for the detection of weak carcinogens and mutagens. In mutagenicity testing even alkylating agents
and other strong mutagens must be given at high doses to yield consis
tent results. At low doses their mutagenic effect is often missed.
It is thus not likely that weak mutagens would be recognized by routine testing. It would be better, therefore, to concentrate on the
few drugs scheduled for commercial introduction and to perform an
exhaustive assessment of their genetic effects in many tests, including in vitro systems. As to carcinogenicity, recent experience has
shown that such effects are often only present in one special strain
of animals. Apart from the questionable significance of such findings, these observations show that a routine carcinogenicity test in
one strain of mice could easily miss other pertinent effects. Here
again, it appears much more reasonable to explore carefully the carcinogenic potential of compounds once they are scheduled for introduction rather than to delay clinical trials of all new candidate
drugs by submitting them to one single long-term rodent experiment
prior to their first use in man.

This problem has most dramatically been highlighted by the recent
controversy about the alleged carcinogenicity of oral contraceptives.
After learning that orally active progestogens caused mammary nodules
in beagle dogs, the US Food and Drug Administration not only stopped
the clinical use of some, but issued far-reaching directives for preclinical safety testing of such compounds (Table 5). The scientific

TABLE 5

FDA Guidelines for Toxicity Testing of Contraceptives,
Estrogens, and Progestogens (from Goldenthal, 1969)

Extent of Clinical Study	Animal Toxicity Study Requirements
Few subjects up to 10 days administration (Phase 1)	90-day studies in rats, dogs, and monkeys
Approximately 50 subjects for 3 menstrual cycles (Phase 2)	1 year studies in rats, dogs, and monkeys
Clinical trial (Phase 3)	2 year studies in rats, dogs, and monkeys. Initiation of 7-year dog and 10-year monkey studies prior to start of Phase 3.
New drug application (Application for marketing)	Up-to-date progress reports on long-term dog and monkey studies

justification of this testing procedure is debatable. Its frustra-
ting impact on the drug industry's effort to slow down overpopulation
was discussed by Djerassi (1969), one of the pharmaceutical manufacturers most outspoken representatives.

The story of the oral contraceptives demonstrates the conflict
between the understandable desire to protect the public against even

the remotest hazard and the urgent necessity to develop therapeutic agents. A satisfactory scientific basis on which to make a just decision is rarely available. For the time being certain guiding principles must therefore be developed which should minimize the risk to the patients without hampering unduly the development of important new drugs:

TABLE 6

Guiding Principles of WHO Scientific Groups for the Selection of Drugs for Carcinogenicity (1969) and Mutagenicity (1971) Testing

A. CARCINOGENIC EFFECTS

1. To Be Tested Before Clinical Trials

   a) Drugs whose chemical structure and biological activities resemble those of known carcinogens or which form metabolites similar to those formed by known carcinogens.

   b) Drugs affecting rapidly growing tissues and mitosis.

2. To Be Tested During Clinical Trials

   Drugs which are administered for long periods of time or to newborn babies, pregnant and lactating women.

3. To be Tested After the Decision to Release for Marketing

   All drugs for which a carcinogenic hazard cannot be ruled out with reasonable confidence.

B. MUTAGENIC EFFECTS

1. To Be Tested Prior to Clinical Trials

   Drugs chemically, biochemically and pharmacologically related to known or suspected mutagens.

2. To Be Tested Prior to Extended Clinical Trials (Phase 3)

   a) Drugs showing certain toxic effects, e.g., depression of hematopoiesis, spermatogenesis and oogenesis, stimulate or inhibit growth of organs, cells or viruses or inhibit immune responses.

   b) Compounds belonging to a new chemical class.

3. To Be Tested After the Decision to Release for Marketing*

   a) Drugs that are used over periods of years, particularly in children.

   b) Drugs that are prescribed for a large proportion of the population.

   c) Drugs subject to widespread abuse.

   d) Drugs that come in contact with sperms in high concentrations, e.g., vaginal contraceptives, compounds used for sperm preservation.

4. Low Priority for Testing

   All others. A few representative compounds of each chemical group should be tested.

* The report of the Scientific Group does not specifically make this proposal but lists this group of drugs under "high priority" without making any recommendations when they should actually be tested.

1) New drugs should be evaluated considering all available chemical and biological information. Extent and timing of testing is decided using the best scientific judgement. This approach was proposed by WHO Scientific Groups on Carcinogenicity and Mutagenicity Testing of Drugs (1969, 1971). Their main recommendations are listed in Table 6.

2) In early clinical trials number of patients and duration of treatment should be limited to the absolute minimum considered necessary to judge tolerance and efficacy. If preliminary results look promising, carcinogenicity and mutagenicity testing should be initiated so that pertinent information is accumulating while clinical evaluation proceeds.

3) Short term screening tests should be developed and used.

4) No risks should be taken with a new drug for which there is no medical need or whose pharmacological profile does not at least suggest certain hopes that it will make a significant contribution to therapy.

The Menace of False Positive Results

This discussion of the needs for testing drugs as a prerequisite for clinical trials would not be complete without at least mentioning another serious problem: the danger that a valuable compound might not be developed because of positive test results that are of little significance for the drug's later use in man. How many patients would have died if isoniazid had been subjected to carcinogenicity testing prior to clinical trials and if its carcinogenic properties would have convinced a powerful regulatory agency that it was too dangerous to be used in man? Isoniazid is not an isolated example. We have recently witnessed others, e.g., hycanthone, a very valuable schistosomiacide whose clinical use was severely criticized because of positive findings in certain mutagenicity screening tests. After considerable soul-searching by many experts the drug was left on the market for the time being. Another highly active schistosomiacide, SQ 18,506, a nitrofurane was not so lucky. Although it possessed quite low toxicity and caused no tumors in rats, it was carcinogenic in mice. Despite its remarkable therapeutic potential in man, further clinical work had to be discontinued although experimental studies on the remarkable schistosomicidal activity of this compound in animals and on the evaluation of its carcinogenic potential for man is being continued (Welch, 1972, personal communication). Has this decision prevented cancer or condemned patients to lifelong suffering? We shall never know.

As toxicological testing procedures get more extensive and sophisticated and as more potent and more specifically acting drugs will be discovered, more and more potentially harmful effects will be found in the preclinical animal experiments. It will often be very difficult to resolve the risk-benefit equation, particularly for new drugs which have the proven risk demonstrated in the animal test, but have no benefit to their credit, since they never had a chance to be used in patients.

Where Toxicological Guidelines Are Hidden

It is not easy at all to lie one's hand on published guidelines for toxicity testing of drugs. Of the 23 references cited by Hebold in his 1972 review of the testing requirements in various countries, only 2 are accessible in regular scientific journals. The others are reports of expert committees and notifications issued by groups of industry scientists or regulatory agencies. It is not that toxicologists want to keep their rules for themselves, but they probably feel that their guidelines are so preliminary and subject to frequent revision that they prefer to keep them out of the scientific literature. However, the two classical papers on drug toxicology are published. One was written by the group of Lehman et al (1955) of the US Food and Drug Administration, the other by Barnes and Denz (1954). Of more recent date are several short articles and letters by Goldenthal (1966, 1968, 1969) which describe the guidelines of the US Food and Drug Administration. The requirements of the American, British, German, Russian, Swedish and Swiss regulatory agencies, the proposed guidelines of the EEC-Commission and of the European Society for the Study of Drug Toxicity (1965) are summarized and documented in the review paper of Hebold (1972).

For the non-specialist the Technical Reports of WHO Scientific Groups on preclinical testing of drugs for safety (1966), clinical evaluation of drugs (1968), testing of drugs for teratogenicity (1967) and the 2 reports on carcinogenicity (1969) and mutagenicity (1971) testing already mentioned will give an excellent and balanced view of the whole problem, apart from being low-priced and available in most countries of the world. A good summary of teratogenic drug screening was recently published by Tuchmann-Duplessis (1972). My own "research" on guidelines and how they have blossomed in the last 10 years is filed in a Science editorial (1969).

TOWARDS A COMPREHENSIVE AND METHODICAL APPROACH TO TOXICOLOGY

Areas of Toxicological Exaggeration and Neglect

When a toxicologist is given a new drug, he usually knows little or nothing about its toxic properties. But unlike his colleagues in pharmacology who can select the qualities for which to test and are free to neglect others, he cannot afford to miss any significant adverse effect. The omnibus procedure described in the previous chapter was therefore developed in the hope that most toxic qualities of a new drug would sooner or later become manifest. And just to make sure that they would come forth, large numbers of animals, massive overdosage, and indiscriminate laboratory examinations became part of the routine procedure. The major value of this testing system (and it has proven very useful in the past despite its shortcomings) is to detect the direct, i.e. specific, toxic effects. These drug reactions, if demonstrable at all, are usually found in most animals treated. Other untoward reactions, however, cannot readily be demonstrated in these experiments (Zbinden, 1964). This is particularly true for those which occur only in a small percentage of patients treated. Even if one assumes similar susceptibility of test animals and man, the chances of finding such untoward reactions in a single subject are slim indeed. Our calculation shown in Table 7 emphasizes this point. Moreover, the fact that a certain toxic drug effect is only seen in a small percentage of patients at risk is generally due to the inhomogeneity of the human population. Only rarely would comparable aberrations occur in the animal kingdom. Even gross exaggerations in the experimental design are therefore not likely to improve significantly the predictability of toxicity tests.

TABLE 7

NUMBER OF ANIMALS IN TOXICITY EXPERIMENTS

Probability of toxic effects in man	Animals in Experiments *	
	Probability 0.95	Probability 0.99
100	1	1
80	2	3
60	4	6
50	5	7
40	6	10
20	14	21
10	29	44
5	59	90
2	149	228
1	299	459
0.1	2'995	4'603
0.01	29'956	46'050
0.001	299'572	------

* Number of animals to be included in experiment in order to find at least one subject with the toxic effect (assuming identical incidence of toxic effect in animals and man). (Calculated by T. Marthaler, Biostatistics Center, University of Zurich)

The inherent insufficiencies of routine toxicity experiments have often been decried, so for example by Barnes and Denz who, in 1954, felt angry enough to write the following statement:

"A chronic toxicity test is always a makeshift affair to be replaced as soon as possible by a more permanent structure of knowledge built on the foundations of physiology, bio-chemistry and other fundamental sciences."

Despite such warnings, routine procedures have grown more rapidly than the practice of using test methods based on fundamental sciences. For many toxic effects such methods are not even available. For others, e.g., various changes of the hormonal balance and disturbance of behavior, useful assay procedures are known. But they are rarely employed by toxicologists, perhaps because their days are filled with the enormous task of satisfying the growing requirements of regulatory agencies for routine toxicity data. Take, for example, the problem of thrombogenic effects of drugs. Despite the great concern that chemical substances might facilitate thrombo-embolism, animal toxicity tests as performed routinely include only rudimentary assay procedures aimed at evaluating the coagulation system. There are, however, many drug effects which could shift the balance of the hemostatic system towards hypercoagulation or impending thrombosis without ever producing thrombo-embolic manifestations in a chronic feeding experiment. Among these are increased tendency of platelets to adhere to foreign surfaces and to aggregate, activation of contact factors, acceleration of various steps of the clotting reaction, reduction of antithrombin III, inhibition of fibrinolysis, increase of free fatty acids, decrease of serum albumin leading to reduced binding of free fatty acids and other substances likely to be involved in thrombus formation, changes of the blood vessel intima, etc. Many of these changes can be assayed in simple animal screening tests. We have learned about them through intensive studies of the potential thrombogenic effect of oral contraceptives. Would it not be better to apply this knowledge routinely, rather than to conduct animal studies of many years duration which have a poor chance of yielding useful information about the thrombogenic potential of new drugs?

This then is one problem in the vast field of toxicological neglect. The reason that there are many more lies in the fact that toxicologists do not often ask specific questions. They prefer to feed the drug and wait to see what happens. But recent research has proven that it pays to ask questions and to tailor the experimental approach in such a way that a reasonable answer can be expected. Assessment of teratogenic and mutagenic risks, evaluation of hepatotoxic and neurotoxic activities, demonstration of psychological dependence in self injection experiments, and the study of the mechanism of drug-induced hemolytic anemias are only a few of many encouraging examples.

Toxicological Check-List for New Drugs

The aim of a comprehensive toxicological evaluation is to learn as much as possible about one's new drug, to relate all biological properties to dose or concentrations, to determine the likelihood that the observed biological effect could be of clinical significance, and to define the circumstances of use which would favor the development of a harmful drug effect in man. This approach is in sharp contrast to the old-fashioned philosophy which considered a toxicological evaluation as an exercise to be done to demonstrate the absence of harmful effects.

For the convenience of drug investigators a check-list is presented in Table 8. It contains a selection of qualities most of which can be readily measured. They are the elements on which the safety evaluation has to rely. The table also includes a number of parameters which modify the drug's action and make it either more toxic or reduce its potential hazards. Not all measurable qualities are equally important and not all need to be known when the compound is first given to man. The importance of the information is therefore rated as follows:

A: Essential for all drugs, to be known before first clinical trial

B: Essential for certain types of drugs, to be known before first clinical trials

C: Very desirable, to be known before or during early clinical trials

D: To be investigated during clinical trials

E: To be investigated in selected cases during clinical trials or after commercial introduction; particularly if suspected from clinical observations or theoretical considerations

TABLE 8

Selected, Important Sources of Toxicological Information

Chemical and Physical

Chemical Structure	A	p K	A
Chemically related drugs	A	Organic solvent-water partition coefficient	A
Stability at various pH	A	Solubility in water and urine at various pH	A
Chemistry of decomposition prod.	D		
Chelating properties	D	Water solubility of major metabolites	D
Photochemical properties and stability	E	Oxidizing properties	C
Surface activity	D	Binding with DNA, RNA, lipids and other macromolecules	E
Binding with serum proteins	C		

Pharmaceutical Formulation

Chemical composition	D	Rate of release of active drug	D

Absorption, Distribution, Metabolism, Excretion

Absorption for all routes of clinically anticipated administration	A	Modification of absorption by pharmaceutical manipulations and nutritional factors	D
Chemical alterations of drug by intestinal flora	E	Penetration through biological membranes (blood-brain, placenta, aqueous humor, etc.)	D
Penetration through normal and inflamed skin	B		
Distribution in body water	D	Tissue distribution incl. fetus	C
Binding and storage in specific tissues, cells or cell components	E	Excretion in milk	D
		Blood and tissue levels after single and repeated administration	C
Sites of metabolism	C	Chemical identity of major metabolites	D
Half-life of active drug and major metabolites in blood and major target organs	C	Modification of metabolism due to various diseases	E
Major pathways of excretion	A	Renal clearance of drug and metabolites	D
Effect on urinary pH	C	Change of excretion by damaged organs	D
Ability to induce or inhibit drug metabolizing microsomal enzymes	A	Effect on conjugation mechanisms	D
Metabolism in newborn animals	D	Ease of removal by peritoneal dialysis	E

Drug Interactions

Modifications of pharmacological effects of drugs likely to be used in combination	D	Potentiation of ethanol, barbiturates and inhalation anesthetics	D
Effect on ethanol metabolism	E	Potential toxicity in combination with enzyme inhibitors	E
Effect on metabolism and anti-coagulant action of coumarin anticoagulants	D	Ability to displace bilirubin and selected drugs from albumin binding sites	D
Competition with other drugs for microsomal metabolizing enzymes	E	Interactions with other modes of therapy	E

In Vitro Investigations

Effect on selected enzymes (carboanhydrase, monoaminoxidase, Krebs-cycle, etc.)	E	Mitochondrial respiration	D
		Cytotoxicity in mammalian cells	D
		Chemotactic motility of leukocytes	E
Phagocytic activity of leukocytes	E	Platelet adhesion and aggregation	E
Osmotic and mechanic red cell fragility	C	Effect on 6-GPD deficient red cells	E
		Isolated organs (heart, atrium, uterus, etc.)	E

Pharmacological Investigations

Central and peripheral neuro-toxicity	C	EEG	C
		Convulsant action	C
Interactions with known convulsants	E	Behavioral toxicity	D
Learning and memory	E	Sexual behavior	E
Physical and psychological dependence	D	Withdrawal effects	D
		Effects on sensory organs	D
Neuromuscular function	D	Extrapyramidal reactions	E
Eating and drinking behavior	D	Blood pressure and regulating mechanisms	A
ECG	A		
Cardiac function	C	Intraocular pressure	D
Pulmonary pressure	D	Various respiratory parameters	D
Regional blood flow	E	Cholinergic and anticholinergic effects	C
Adrenergic and adrenolytic effects	C		
Gastric secretion	D	Gastrointestinal ulcers	D
Gastrointestinal motility	D	Emetic effects	E
Liver function	A	Interference with absorption of nutrients	E
Bile flow	D		
Intrabiliary pressure	E	Kidney function	A
Diuretic effects	C	Body temperature	A

Intermediary Metabolism

Basal metabolic rate	C	Fasting blood sugar and glucose load	C
Insulin release	E	Insulin sensitivity	E
Free fatty acid mobilization	D	Blood and liver lipids	D
Cholesterol synthesis	E	Liver triglyceride secretion	E
Protein synthesis	D	Serum proteins	C
Aminoaciduria	D	Bilirubin and bile acid metabolism	D
Oxalate metabolism	D	Synthesis, storage and release of biogenetic amines	D
Uric acid formation and excretion	E		
Water and electrolyte balance	C	Vitamin metabolism	E
Porphyrin metabolism	E	Iron metabolism	E

Endocrine Investigations

Pituitary function	E	Pituitary-adrenal axis	D
Estrus cycle	D	Stimulation and inhibition of sex	D
Thyroid function	D	hormone dependent organs	
Parathyroid function	E	Anabolic and anti-anabolic effects	D
Antidiuretic effect	D		

Experimental Pathology

Effect on injured organs	E	Mitosis, growth, differention,	E
Effect on experimental diabetes	E	regeneration	
Inflammatory responses	D	Bacterial, virus and fungus infections	D
Immune reaction, antibody synthesis	D	Complement action	E
Function of reticuloendothelial system	E	Blood coagulation and hemostasis	D
		Fibrinolysis	D
Interaction with stress	E	Red cell and platelet survival	E
Methemoglobin formation	A	Effects on spontaneous diseases	E
Phototoxicity, photosensitivity	E	including tumors	
Interference with diagnostic tests	E	Contact sensitization	B
Experiments with animals having genetic enzyme abnormality	E	Effects of unbalanced diets	E

Toxicity Studies*

Acute toxicity	A	Subacute and chronic toxicity	A-D
Reproduction	C	Teratogenic effects	A-D
Neonatal development	D	Carcinogenic effects	E
Mutagenic effects	A-E	Sensitizing properties (parenteral)	A-E
Local toxicity (skin, eye, vagina, intrathecal, etc)	B		

*   The timing of these studies is discussed in detail on pages 8 - 16.

The check-list is not a complete collection of all sources of toxicological information. And not all its points are essential or even applicable for all types of drugs, but it contains several bits which I have neglected to collect repeatedly and which then had to be gathered in a hurry. It is hoped that it will help others to avoid such embarrassment.

A similar but more voluminous check-list should be used for the clinical evaluation of the side-effect liability of new drugs. It is not wise to wait for the first patient to fall down the staircase before making the necessary effort to look for orthostatic hypotension with appropriate procedures. Thus, clinical trials should not merely register side-effects as they happen but should be designed to assess frequency and dose-dependency of adverse effects. Apart from providing important clinical information, such studies will be most valuable for the toxicologist who depends on clinical feedback for the evaluation of the toxicological assay procedures.

ACUTE TOXICITY

Measurement

The most popular way to describe the acute toxic qualities of a drug is to list its median lethal doses (LD_{50}) in various species. As a matter of fact, the determination of the LD_{50} is, without any doubt, the most frequently performed pharmacological experiment. It is a ritual mass execution of animals and is done as follows: The laboratory animals, usually small rodents, are starved overnight or longer. Groups of 10 or more of both sexes are then treated once with the test drug. Doses have to be chosen so that some animals of at least 3 groups succumb within an observation period of at least 7 days. From the number of dead a dose is calculated which would presumably kill 50% of the animals.

Note that the determination of the LD_{50} is based on an all or none response and each animal is only used once. (Re-use of survivors for a new test is advocated by parsimonious pharmacologists, but it has not become common practice). All or none responses are the statistician's delight. Consequently, they have come forward with ever more brilliant refinements of their computation methods, best described in Finney's (1964) classical treatise on the biological assay. The standard procedure is that of Bliss (1935) and Fisher (1935). For practical purposes toxicologists usually determine the LD_{50} with graphic methods. Those of Litchfield and Wilcoxon (1949), Miller and Tainter (1944), and DeBeer (1945) have the most devotees. Others recommend computing methods whose advantages and disadvantages are discussed by Cornfield and Mantel (1950).

Importance of Experimental Conditions

The LD_{50} of a drug is dependent on age, sex, weight and genetic background of the animals, duration of the starvation period prior to dosing, ambient temperature, concentration of the test substances, speed of injection, and type of solvent or suspension medium. Toxicologists using pathogen-free animals are often rewarded with higher LD_{50}'s. Also important is the number of animals per cage: crowding greatly increases the toxicity of stimulants. From this enumeration of factors affecting the LD_{50}, it is clear that the experimental conditions must be carefully controlled. But if this is done, the variability can be kept to a minimum, even if experiments are performed in different, professionally supervised laboratories (Weil and Wright, 1967). In this way the precise determination of the LD_{50} can serve as a convenient and sensitive analytical tool which recognizes toxic impurities and physical and chemical changes affecting bioavailability.

What LD_{50} Figures Are Used For

For new drugs regulatory agencies require LD_{50}'s with at least 2 animal species and 2 routes of administration. Some toxicologists will do much better than that and obtain LD_{50} values of any animal species and strain within their reach. Should one not better stop and think what this considerable effort really contributes to the safety evaluation of a new drug? The LD_{50} figures as such permit nothing more than a preliminary classification of the poisonousness of a substance. Environmental toxicologists have developed a toxicity rating system which is strictly based on mortality. Although they prefer to establish this classification using the probable lethal dose for a 70 kg man, they will substitute the LD_{50}'s obtained in experimental animals if human data are not available. The 6 toxicity classes so determined are listed in Table 9. Most drugs are neither supertoxic nor harmless and are to be found in class 4 (e.g., caffeine, chlorpromazine, aspirin) or class 5 (e.g., amphetamine). Thus, they are considerably more dangerous than your favorite whisky, rated class 2 (Gleason et al., 1969).

TABLE 9

Toxicity Rating*

Toxicity Class		Probable Lethal Dose for a 70 kg Man** mg/kg
6	supertoxic	less than 5
5	extremely toxic	5-50
4	very toxic	50-500
3	moderately toxic	500-5,000
2	slightly toxic	5,000-15,000
1	practically nontoxic	above 15,000

*   From Gleason et al., 1969

** Lacking human data, it is a conventional assumption that the LD_{50} of test animals can be substituted for the mean lethal dose in man.

There is no consistent relationship between the LD_{50} and chronic toxicity, since the cause of death occurring after a single high dose may be entirely different from that encountered after repeated administration of subtoxic doses. It follows that the frequently used procedure to take a certain fraction of the LD_{50} as a basis for chronic experiments can lead to costly surprises. Peck (1968) tells about one he experienced with dexamethasone which had a s.c. LD_{50} (7 day observation) in rats of 120 mg/kg but was not tolerated by rats and dogs at daily doses of more than 0.07 mg/kg.

Other Toxicological Aspects

With a modest effort the LD_{50} determination can yield much useful additional information. Particularly instructive is the observation of symptoms preceding death. It not only permits certain conclusions regarding mechanism of action but also provides important background information on what might happen should the new drug (as it certainly will) be misused for a suicidal attempt. Valuable hints about the main target organs of the new drug could also be obtained through systematic autopsy of animals dying during acute toxicity experiments. Traditionally such autopsies are rarely performed and important information is lost. On the other hand, histopathological examination of the organs is not recommended as a routine procedure. Although interesting findings might emerge, the organ changes of animals dying from acute overdosage are so ambiguous that an intelligent assessment would be difficult. Moreover, the information likely to be gained over that furnished by gross observation would only occasionally justify the additional technical effort. I would not be surprised, however, if future research would compel me to revise this statement.

What must be observed carefully in an LD_{50} experiment is the time of death. In general animals die 2-24 hrs after single high doses. But sometimes survival time is only a few minutes or less. In such cases an acute pharmacological effect such as depression of the respiratory center or cardiac function, convulsions, or deep narcosis may be the cause of death. Drugs inducing such dramatic responses at high doses may nevertheless be tolerated over long periods of time if the dose is kept at a level causing less than the maximal pharmacological effect. These compounds are often characterized by a steep dose-effect curve. This is another reason why they are difficult to handle and can be dangerous for the careless patient. Thus, the poisonousness of a drug should not only be judged from its LD_{50} figure but also from the slope of the dose-effect curve.

A survival time of 1 to 2 weeks is often found in acute toxicity experiments with drugs causing bone marrow depression and injury of the intestinal mucosa. For example: the oral LD_{50} of cyclophosphamide in rats was 720 mg/kg after 2 days of observation, 235 mg/kg after 5 days and was down to 94 mg/kg after 14 days (Wheeler et al., 1962). Animals treated with corticosteroids died even later, due to slowly progressing infections and abscess formation. Triamcinolone had a s.c. LD_{50} in rats of 864 mg/kg if calculated after 1 week of observation, but it decreased to 99 mg/kg over a period of three more weeks (Tonelli, 1966).

If the oral LD_{50} is much higher than that found after parenteral administration, poor enteral absorption or destruction of the drug in the gut must be suspected. In such cases the LD_{50} experiment will give quick information about the possibility of improving absorbtion by pharmaceutical manipulations.

A rare but interesting finding in LD_{50} determinations is the polyphasic dose-effect curve. It was described for, among others, DL-amphetamine. With this agent the i.p. lethality in mice increased between 15 and 45 mg/kg, decreased from 45-75 mg/kg and increased again at doses over 75 mg/kg. Such effects can only be found if experiments are performed with doses narrowly spaced. They suggest the presence of 2 or more different actions of the drug contributing to the lethal effect (Gardocki et al., 1966).

From this discussion it is clear that for the toxicologist, and certainly also for the clinical pharmacologist, the numerical value of the LD_{50} as such is of much less importance than the many additional observations to be made during the acute toxicity experiments. Give them this additional information and they are (or should be) satisfied with an approximate LD_{50} value. This figure is sufficient to classify the new drug within the overall toxicity rating system.

All further conclusions as to mechanism of action, main target organs and clinical significance are derived essentially from clinical observations. These, however, can be gained with a much smaller effort and fewer animals. Some of the simplified methods worked out in the past are described below. They are adequate for many purposes and should not be sacrificed to an unnecessary craving for perfectionism. This is particularly important when we work with larger animals whose death must give us much more than just a terribly precise LD_{50} figure. Here are, in brief, some of these alternate testing procedures:

The Up-and-Down Method uses somewhat fewer animals than the conventional LD_{50}-determination but gives equally exact data. It was introduced by Dixon and Mood (1948) who developed it for the assay of sensitivity of explosives to shock. It provides for a sequential treatment of animals starting with a dose estimated to be close to the median lethal dose. The following animal is given a higher dose if the first survives, or a lower dose, if it has died. As a consequence, most animals are treated with doses near the true mean lethal dose. This improves accuracy of the statistical calculation and reduces the number of animals needed. A disadvantage of the method is the necessity to treat the animals sequentially. Since it takes much longer for an animal to die than for an explosive to detonate, an LD_{50} determination will require much time. This problem can largely be avoided if the modified procedure of Brownlee et al. (1953) is used.

The Approximate Lethal Dose Method claimed by its inventors Deichmann and LeBlanc (1943) to require approximately six animals goes as follows: 6 animals are treated once and simultaneously with doses each of which is 50% higher than the preceding one. This spacing of doses is sufficient to preclude the possibility of killing one animal with a dose while failing to kill the animal with the next higher dose. In this way it is possible to determine the smallest lethal dose which, as experience shows, is close to the LD_{50}. Exploring this range-finding test on 87 compounds, Deichmann and Mergard (1948) found that 88% of the approximate lethal doses ranged within ± 30% of the respective LD_{50}'s obtained with considerably higher cost. This may seem quite a large variation, but looking at their original figures, it is interesting to note that the range finding procedure permitted correct toxicity ratings in all but very few of the compounds tested.

Another useful range finding procedure is that proposed by E. A. Maynard who described it briefly in the paper of Smith et al. (1960). A unit dose (ml,mg,g) is arbitrarily selected and injected into 2 mice. After 24 hrs a second pair of mice is treated using a factor of 3/2 if the first dose was tolerated or 2/3 if it was fatal. This procedure is continued until the maximal non-lethal and the minimal lethal doses are known. If the initial guess was not too far off, it should not take many mice to reach this goal. All additional observations, i.e., major toxic symptoms, main target organ, survival time, can, of course, also be made.

An excellent procedure for estimation of median lethal doses is based on the method of moving averages described by Thompson (1947). It can be used, as Smyth et al. (1962) showed with very few animals. Prerequisites are: a constant number of animals per dosage level whereby this number can be as low as 2, spacing of dosage levels in a geometric progression and a certain minimal number of dose levels. Instead of fitting the data to complex mathematical curves, the moving average method takes the arithmetic means of 3 successive values of percent dead animals and relates them to the mean of the corresponding doses. By simple computations the LD_{50} and the 95% confidence interval can be determined. But best of all, Weil (1952) has published tables which permit an even simpler calculation of these values. Furthermore, he has shown that LD_{50} results with 30 compounds were, with one exception, practically the same as those obtained with the classical method of Bliss (1935). I cannot hide my prejudice for Weil's tables and formulas but must admit at the same time that my preference is motivated by their simplicity and not by any deep insight into the intricacies of statistical argumentation.

Finally, it should be stressed that an acute toxicity test does not necessarily imply single dose treatment. Treating animals, particularly large animals, every day or every other day with doubling doses will provide a wealth of information as long as the appropriate clinical and laboratory observations are made. Instead of the LD_{50} one gains information about the minimal symptomatic and the minimal toxic dose, major symptoms of intoxication, principal target organs, duration of drug action, and reversibility of toxic injuries. Show me the clinical pharmacologist who would ask for more!

III

SPECULATIVE TOXICOLOGY

GENERAL REMARKS

As drugs are absorbed and distributed with the blood stream and
as they penetrate through biological membranes and enter all compart-
ments biochemical pharmacologists can dream of, a large number of
chemical reactions takes place. Only a minority of them will be no-
ticed either by a lessening of bothersome symptoms or by the emer-
gence of new disturbing subjective signs of discomfort. Few of the
chemical interactions between drugs and living matter produce measurable biochemical or functional changes and only occasionally do they
cause morphological alterations. But whatever drugs do and wherever
they go, once they have performed their intended function, they are
no more wanted and are potentially harmful. Scientists like to speculate about the toxicological implications of every aspect of a drug's
contacts with the organism. Very often their investigations and
speculations open up entangled problems which are more difficult to
sort out than it was originally believed. A certain friend of mine
used to liken the speculative toxicologist to the small boy on a
fishing trip who, after opening an innocent-looking can of worms,
must spend all his precious time trying to put those worms back into
the can. Many a scientist has used his time trying to solve an
equally elusive problem of speculative toxicology. Others, however,
have been successful, and if they have not resolved all the problems
they set out to conquer, they have certainly added new and exciting
dimensions to drug toxicology which, without their work, might have
become a slightly stale branch of biological sciences.

INDUCTION OF DRUG METABOLIZING ENZYMES

Experimental Background

The discovery of the microsomal drug metabolizing enzymes has
stimulated toxicological research like few events before. A group of
enzymes thought to play only a modest role in endogenous steroid
metabolism, was for a long time, neglected by most biochemists. It
suddenly reached the center of attention when it was realized that it
helped the body to eliminate those lipid soluble chemicals which were
nowhere in sight when evolution and natural selection determined the
composition of our enzymatic make-up. The fact that the working of
this biochemical detoxification mechanism could be demonstrated in
simple but convincing, indeed often dramatic, mouse and rat experiment

contributed much to the biochemists enthusiasm. So much so, that several of their best were subsequently won over to toxicology.

After a few injections of an inducing substance, rats and mice respond with an impressive synthesis of microsomal liver enzymes. Metabolism of lipid soluble drugs is greatly enhanced which can be readily demonstrated by certain standard experiments, e.g., shortening of narcosis induced by 75-150 mg/kg hexobarbital i.p., inhibition of paralysis following injection of 150 mg/kg zoxazolamine or a rapid elimination of aminopyrine from the blood (Conney et al., 1960, Hansen and Fouts, 1968). At autopsy one finds an enlarged liver with disappointing histopathological changes such as centrolobular swelling and reduced basophilia of the cytoplasm. In the electron microscope preparation the marked increase of the smooth endoplasmatic reticulum is impressive (Remmer and Merker, 1963). In the microsomal fraction of the liver, a distinct increase in oxidative, reducing, demethylating, hydroxylating and conjugating enzyme activities can readily be demonstrated. Nuclear RNA polymerase is activated (Gelboin et al., 1967) and ascorbic acid excretion in the urine is markedly increased (Hoogland et al., 1966). Typically, most of these changes are inhibited by CCl_4 and ethionine treatment. Not all drugs stimulate all the above-named enzymatic reactions. Possible explanations for these differences and their pharmacological implications were extensively reviewed by Conney (1967). Gillette (1971) and others have added exciting insight into the molecular basis of this important biological mechanism.

Enzyme stimulation is not an exclusive privilege of the liver. It occurs also in other tissues, notably the lung, gastrointestinal tract, and kidney. Nevertheless, most experiments focus on the liver of the rat where the events proceed with such ease that one is tempted to work with this organ only. Just feeding rats with charcoal broiled hamburgers in which minute amounts of polycyclic hydrocarbons are formed is enough to induce their liver enzymes (Harrison and West, 1971). But keep in mind that in this field of biology species differences are most important. For example, the liver of primates including man is normally rich in endoplasmatic reticulum, and it is therefore most difficult to find a morphological substrate of drug-induced enzyme stimulation. Furthermore, remarkable quantitative and qualitative species differences not only with regard to enzyme activity but also to chemical composition of the microsomal subfractions have been recognized (Gram et al., 1971).

The review of Conney (1967) names many of the known enzyme-stimulating substances. Here are just a few of the important ones: among the most active are insecticides, such as chlordane, DDT and hexachlorocyclohexene; furthermore, barbiturates, phenylbutazone, tolbutamide and the polycyclic hydrocarbons 3-methylcholanthrene and 3,4-benzpyrene. Ethanol, ether, chlordiazepoxide, steroid hormones and laughing gas are examples for weak inducers.

Toxicological Implications

The central importance of the microsomal enzyme system for the elimination of a large proportion of currently used drugs has naturally invited speculations about its role as a toxicological mechanism. That this endeavor has perhaps not yielded as much incriminating evidence as some may have hoped, is due to the fact that the system's most important function is that of detoxification and getting rid of unnatural chemicals. True, if one is a rat or a dog and is forced to have one's liver enzymes stimulated by repeated injections of high doses of phenobarbital, various undesired reactions can take place: the metabolism of other drugs such as diphenylhydantoin is accelerated so that therapeutic levels are no longer reached. On the other hand, a compound given at high doses and possessing strong binding affinity to the enzyme protein may competitively inhibit the metabolism of another drug. For such an action watch chloramphenicol (Grogan et al. 1972) which is normally given at rather high doses and can prolong the half life of tolbutamide, diphenylhydantoin and dicoumarol and may in this way be responsible for an exaggeration of their pharmacological and toxic effects. Such an enzyme inhibition must, however, not necessarily be competitive, but the inhibitors can in some other way act on membranes and enzyme proteins. Thus several drugs, hydrazines for example (Kato et al., 1969) have been found to inhibit drug metabolizing enzymes. It is not unreasonable, therefore, to insist on knowing what a new drug does to microsomal enzymes before it is released for wide clinical use.

A drug may stimulate its own metabolism so much that it ceases to be pharmacologically active (Burns et al., 1967). An example is tolbutamide whose blood level in dogs may drop as much as 80% on continued administration with concomitant development of tolerance for the hypoglycemic effect (Welch et al., 1967). Another toxicological lesson is learned from the dicoumarol-treated dog that also receives barbiturates and whose anticoagulant dose must be increased to maintain the desired prolongation of prothrombin time. If the barbiturate medication is discontinued, enzyme stimulation is reduced and dicoumarol metabolism slows down. As a consequence, severe hypoprothrombinemia with hemorrhage may ensue (Conney and Burns, 1972).

Certain chemicals must be activated in the liver to form a poisonous metabolite. In animals with stimulated microsomal enzymes this activation proceeds at a faster rate and toxicity becomes more severe. The best example is that of carbon tetrachloride and related halogenated hydrocarbons. These are apparently metabolized to very reactive epoxides in the centrolobular liver cells, form covalent bonds with macromolecules and destroy the cells. In phenobarbital-pretreated animals liver damage becomes more disastrous than in normal controls (Stenger et al., 1970; Brodie et al., 1971). A similar mechanism operates with organophosphorus insecticides. Some, e.g., dimethoate, undergo enzymatic activation by liver microsomes and consequently are much more toxic in animals with stimulated drug metabolizing enzymes. Other compounds of the same group, however, are more rapidly detoxified in the liver of enzyme-stimulated animals which become more resistant against their harmful effects (Conney, 1967, Menzer and Best, 1968). This is not the only example of a beneficial action of enzyme stimulation. Rats which receive single high doses of phenylbutazone for example will, if their liver enzymes were previously stimulated, metabolize the compound so rapidly that the acute toxic effect, gastric ulcers, does not develop (Burns et al., 1967). Moreover, even the cancer-inducing action of certain chemical carcinogens may be abolished due to a rapid detoxification and elimination of the dangerous substance by the activated liver enzymes of a drug-pretreated animal (Conney, 1967). So whether our rat is better or worse off with stimulated microsomal enzymes depends largely on the chemical nature of the additional substances forced on him during his career as a toxicological subject.

There are several reasons why toxicological speculations from these very elegant experiments should be tempered with caution. First of all, the demonstrative experiments often work only if enzyme induction is forced by high doses of the inducing drug and when the subsequent challenge with another agent is limited to a single administration. When the circumstances of the experiment are changed, the results may be quite confusing. Furthermore, toxicological experiments on the significance of enzyme induction have uncovered a host of species, strain and sex differences (Fujii et al., 1968, Page and Vesell, 1969) as well as other modifying influences such as age, diet, route of administration, altitude, hormonal changes, etc. Gillette (1971) has discussed the possible molecular mechanisms of these factors and the toxicologist must keep them in mind when he attempts to extrapolate the findings in animals to the clinical situation in man. But he should also remember that his own chronic toxicity studies fulfill all requirements for microsomal enzyme induction: They are conducted with high doses over prolonged periods of time and in many instances, this treatment may stimulate liver enzymes to such an extent that severely toxic levels of the drug will never be reached. This is another reason why the action of a new drug on liver enzymes must be known as soon as extended experimental and clinical work is contemplated.

Significance for Man

That enzyme induction can occur in man was demonstrated beyond doubt by biochemical investigations: Antipyrine and phenylbutazone metabolism was found to be accelerated in workers of an insecticide (DDT, Lindane) plant (Kolmodin et al., 1969, Conney et al., 1971). Barbiturate medication, just as in the dog, decreased the half-life of diphenylhydantoin in the blood of epileptic patients. And all clinicians are familiar with the problem of the cardiac patient returning home from the hospital where he was stabilized on an oral anticoagulant. Not needing the barbiturate hypnotic anymore which he was given nightly at the ward, he stops stimulating his mixed function oxydases and may experience severe hemorrhage due to reduced metabolism of the coumarin anticoagulant.

Competitive inhibition of metabolism of a lipid soluble drug by another compound can also occur in man. Diphenylhydantoin detoxification for example can be inhibited by bishydroxycoumarin with an increase of the anticonvulsant's blood level of 250% and a prolongation of its half-life in the blood from 9 hrs up to 44 hrs. No wonder that under these conditions diphenylhydantoin intoxications have developed (Hansen et al., 1966).

Directions for Further Toxicological Speculations

Despite a seemingly clear-cut case clinicians do not seem overly concerned about toxicological implications of microsomal enzyme induction. They acknowledge that due to various interactions the metabolism of a drug can be increased or slowed down. But it appears that these variations are rarely of such a magnitude that they could not be handled by adjustment of the dose. It should not be forgotten that the availability of various dosage forms and the freedom of prescribing a dose depending on the patient's response gives the physician a great versatility with which to overcome changes in metabolic rate of drugs. The patient frequently introduces huge variations of his own by missing one or several doses or by taking more than the prescribed amount if the desired effect is not obtained. Clearly, the problem of enzyme induction is one of the low potency-high dosage chemicals. It is not unnecessary molecular manipulation, therefore, when pharmaceutical chemists try to replace these agents with the more potent congener, a drug which does the same as the previous one but does it with fewer molecules and with less strain on the smooth endoplasmatic reticulum.

More toxicological speculations, however, are needed about the subtle effects of enzyme induction. Recent studies have indicated that animals and human subjects may present distinct changes of the endogenous steroid metabolism if they are chronically exposed to stimulants of drug metabolizing enzymes. There are quantitative shifts in metabolism of androgens, estrogens, progesterone, and corticosteroids resulting in an accelerated hydroxylation of steroid hormones (Conney, 1967). In enzyme stimulated rats, the uterotropic effect of exogenous estrogens was found to be reduced (Levin et al., 1968). How will such changes affect various physiological regulations? How will, for example, the inflammatory response be affected? Experiments have shown a dramatic reduction in response of the peritoneum to the irritant effect of phenylbutazone in animals with phenobarbital pretreatment (Zbinden, 1966a). Is such a modification of an important reactive mechanism of the body good, bad, or meaningless? Another question: Is an enzymatically stimulated, swollen liver a healthy organ prepared to respond to noxious stimuli such as a drinking bout, a halothane narcosis, a virus infection? Can enzyme stimulation be used therapeutically when activation of protein synthesis in the liver or increased detoxification of a foreign chemical is desirable? What is the meaning of enzyme induction in the placenta (Conney et al., 1971) and how does it affect the unborn child? Are some people more likely to respond to enzyme stimulators? Recent evidence indicates that this is probably the case and that the response of the microsomal enzymes is under genetic control (Vesell and Page, 1968; Conney et al., 1971). One enzyme in particular, aryl hydrocarbon hydroxylase (benzpyrene hydroxylase), has recently attracted much attention, since its induction by polycyclic hydrocarbons is inherited as a simple autosomal dominant trait in mice. It is present in C57 BL/6N inbred mice but not in several other strains (Nebert et al., 1972). Do similar inherited differences exist in man? Do these facts hide a clue to the problem of unusual toxic reactions occurring only in a small percentage of the patients and what is their significance for chemical carcinogenesis? The ability to study induction of aryl hydrocarbon hydroxylase in cultured human cells from the foreskins of circumcised babies (Levin et al., 1972) or phytohemagglutinin-stimulated leukocytes (Busbee et al., 1972) may soon lead to highly interesting answers.

The references cited indicate that toxicologists are abandoning, perhaps regretfully, the elegant rat and mouse experiments with 3 days phenobarbital pretreatment and single high dose challenge with another lipid soluble drug. There are more important problems waiting, such

as the questions of what chronic, lifelong exposure to enzyme stimulants means for the ability of man to cope with environmental chemicals and how these subtle changes can be assessed in the human
population. Anybody interested in these questions will be greatly
helped by the authoritative treatise of Conney and Burns (1972) in
which the interaction of environmental chemicals and drugs are extensively discussed.

PROTEIN BINDING

Basic Facts

Many drugs bind reversibly to proteins; first, of course, to
those of the blood. Of the plasma proteins the albumins carry the
greatest load, but macroglobulins, glycoproteins, and other fractions
also participate (Clausen, 1966). There are (there must be) drug-
binding proteins in tissues, but not much is known about their chemical nature.

Albumins have not more than 5 or 6 primary and 20 or more second-
ary binding sites, but generally only 1 or 2 are occupied by drugs
(Thorp, 1964). Much has been speculated about the nature of the binding between drugs and albumin, but the problem, and no one has said
it more eloquently than Brodie (1965), is far from being solved.
Toxicologists and clinical investigators do well to leave this question to the chemists and to accept a few empirical facts: 1) the
fraction of bound drug increases with increasing protein concentration
and decreases when protein concentration is lowered. That means:
when you dilute your serum sample, the degree of protein binding decreases (Anton, 1968). 2) Changing the concentration of the drug has
the opposite effect: the bound fraction is lower with increasing
concentration and higher with decreasing drug levels (Brodie, 1965).
3) The extent of protein binding depends on the chemical structure of
the compound. With sulfonamides, for example, it ranges from 10%
(sulfanilamide) to almost 100% (sulfadimethoxine). It is also in-
fluenced by lipid solubility, high lipid solubility being accompanied
by a high degree of protein binding (Brodie, 1965). 4) The higher the
affinity constant of a drug, the tighter will be the protein binding
and the greater the bound fraction. 5) Protein binding varies with
pH and temperature. 6) Various methods of determination of protein
binding often give differing results (Kunin, 1967). 7) Serum proteins
of different species vary considerably in their ability to bind drugs.
Methotrexate, for example, is bound 40% by dog serum, 50% by mice,
and 65% by rat serum (Dixon et al., 1965). Similar differences were
noted with the basic drug desipramine, which is highly bound by serum
albumins of cats and dogs and much less by rabbit proteins. Human
and rat serums are between the two extremes. (Borga et al., 1968).
8) Published data on albumin concentration in plasma of laboratory
animals may be quite different from those which you find in the blood
of your own animals.

Toxicological Implications

Protein binding is the first and perhaps the most important defense mechanism of the body against injurious effects of drugs and

endogenous substances. Drugs and endogenous substances fight for the available binding sites. Losers remain unattached and are free to penetrate into the tissues. Such interactions may lead to irreparable damage in premature babies whose conjugation and excretion of bilirubin is deficient due to a lack of glucuronyltransferase. If jaundiced babies are given acidic drugs, e.g., sulfonamides or salicylates bilirubin is displaced from albumin binding sites and can penetrate into the brain where it causes deleterious kernicterus. This process can be reproduced experimentally with Gunn strain rats. The homozygous descendents of this strain exhibit the syndrome of non-hemolytic unconjugated hyperbilirubinemia which is also due to a deficiency of glucuronyltransferase. If such animals are injected with sulfonamides salicylates, or caffeine, they quickly perish of kernicterus.

If two drugs compete for protein binding sites, the one with the greater affinity constant will rapidly displace the other. The latter then reaches the tissue receptors at higher concentrations and its pharmacological effects may be exaggerated. A practically important example is warfarin. In the blood only 3% are in the free, active form. The anticoagulant is displaced from its albumin binding sites by many acidic drugs, e.g., diazoxide, mefenamic, nalidixic and ethacrinic acid, phenylbutazone and trichloroacetic acid, a metabolite of chloral hydrate (Sellers and Koch-Weser, 1971). The use of these agents in patients on oral anticoagulants is therefore frequently marred by bleeding episodes. Other examples are the displacement of tolbutamide by sulfonamides and phenylbutazone resulting in acute hypoglycemia (Christensen et al., 1963), and the exaggerated bone marrow depression with ulcerations of mucous membranes if patients on methotrexate therapy are given sulfonamides or salicylates (Dixon et al., 1965). It is also interesting to note that drugs which by themselves have little effect on protein binding can displace a highly bound compound when they are present in combination (Anton, 1968). Protein binding also affects drug metabolism. Unbound drugs are more rapidly detoxified, whereas protein binding, as shown for sulfonamide acetylation, markedly delays the metabolic process (Newbould and Kilpatric, 1960).

Toxicological Speculations

How strong is our first line of defense against foreign chemicals? Looking at our standing army, we can count on an elite corps comprising about 10^{21} albumin molecules and an auxiliary force of other serum proteins and red cells. The carrying capacity of plasma is sufficient for an approximate drug concentration of 7×10^{-4} M. It is perhaps more meaningful to say that a drug with a molecular weight of 280 will have saturated the important albumin binding sites at a plasma level of about 200 μg/ml. (Thorp, 1964) With drugs given in gram quantities, such levels may occasionally be reached or exceeded. Nevertheless, there is a large reservoir of albumin molecules ready to act in our behalf. But do they always report to duty in full numbers and with clean, reactive binding sites? Certainly not! Even in healthy people albumin levels vary from 3.5-5.5 g per 100 ml. Low levels prevail in pregnancy. Moreover, hypalbuminemia is frequent in malnutrition and as a complication of many diseases. Toxicologists know that some drugs, such as L-asparaginase (Haskell et al., 1969) and the estrogen components of oral contraceptives (Adlercreutz et al., 1968), were also found guilty of lowering serum albumin. Any reduction of the albumin levels has a negative effect on the total binding capacity of the blood. As pointed out above, the number of available binding sites may further be reduced because drugs or endogenous chemicals may already have occupied a good part of them.

In every situation a certain percentage of the binding sites is taken by unesterified (free) fatty acids (FFA). These substances invite particularly interesting speculations. They are tightly bound to albumins, but should they ever occur unattached to serum proteins, they reveal themselves as among the most powerful villains our endogenous metabolism can produce. In vitro FFA cause hypercoagulability of the blood (Botti and Ratnoff, 1963), platelet aggregation (Hoak et al., 1966), and platelet damage (Zbinden et al., 1970). It is not surprising, therefore, that widespread thrombosis, particularly in the lung (Zbinden, 1967), pulmonary hypertension, and endothelial damage (Bloom, 1967) occur following i.v. injection into animals. Moreover, cardiotoxic effects of FFA were demonstrated in the isolated heart (Severeid et al., 1969) as well as the intact dog (Connor et al., 1963). It could be due to their uncoupling action on oxidative phosphorylation. All these injurious effects of FFA are abolished if enough albumin binding sites are available. But an excessive release of these acids due to stress or hunger and following the injection of drugs could, at least temporarily, push the FFA levels of the blood above the critical mark of about 1200 µEq/liter. This would provide a molar ratio of FFA to albumin of 2 or more. And that is precisely the ratio at which albumin loses its neutralizing power for FFA in various model systems.

Drugs known to increase serum FFA belong to many different pharmacological classes and act by diverse mechanisms. Among the most active are epinephrine and related compounds, theophylline and caffeine, heparin, ACTH and growth hormone. If FFA are released acutely in the presence of highly protein-bound drugs, an interesting contest will develop; namely, who will displace whom and who will therefore have the first choice to exercise its uninhibited toxic power?

That a suspicious attitude towards the FFA is not without justification is learned from the experiments of Hoak et al. (1963) with ACTH-treated rabbits. In these animals toxic symptomatology and shortened silicone clotting time were clearly related to serum FFA-levels. The autopsy revealed pulmonary thrombosis. Laboratory evidence of hypercoagulability also accompanied raising FFA levels in dogs after injection of caffeine (Bellet et al., 1968). The clinically established observation that obese patients are prone to develop thrombosis after going on a crash diet further supports the notion that highly elevated FFA levels could be an important risk factor. Just as important would be reduced albumin levels and the presence of tightly protein-bound chemical substances. There is also evidence that under pathological conditions, particularly in uremia, serum albumin might be qualitatively altered (Anton and Corey, 1971; Shoeman and Azarnoff, 1972) and thereby further reduce the carrying capacity of an already overtaxed detoxification system.

PYRIDOXAL PHOSPHATE

Biochemical Aspects

An excellent way to start a game of toxicological speculation goes like this: Ask, "What would happen if a drug binds specifically to an important and ubiquitous substance which is essential for survival?" Take any one, for example, vitamin B_6, which is involved in a large variety of metabolic reactions (Holtz and Palm, 1964). To answer, consider that the most important catalytic form of this vitamin is pyridoxal phosphate. Its aldehyde group in position 4 is an easily accessible point of attack for several drugs, resulting in a blockade of coenzyme functions. The metabolic changes of such a blockade are characteristic for vitamin B_6 deficiency, and include increased xanthurenic acid and kynurenine excretion particularly after a tryptophan load, often also increased oxalic and decreased pyridoxic acid excretion (Kang and DaVanzo, 1966). It is probable that such drug-induced disturbance of vitamin B_6 metabolism would express itself in many different ways depending on the tissue distribution of the blocking agent, the affinity of the blocker to the various enzymes, including those not containing pyridoxal phosphate, the availability of alternative metabolic pathways and the organ in which the interaction has taken place. Thus, there is no limit to toxicological speculations.

What Toxicologists Already Know

The most notorious blockers of pyridoxal phosphate are carbonyl-trapping agents, such as hydrazines, semicarbazides, and thiosemicarbazides. They easily penetrate into the brain where the enzymatic perturbation is swiftly converted into dramatic epileptic seizures.

Of the chemicals mentioned, the compound which is medically the most important is isoniazid. It causes convulsions in animals and man as expected, but usually only after gross overdosage. More important for medical practice is its ability to lower the seizure threshold for other convulsant drugs, e.g., metrazol, aminopyrine and procaine even at therapeutic doses (Dienemann and Simon, 1953). For reasons not clarified as yet, the neurotoxic effects of isoniazid manifest themselves particularly in axonal degeneration of peripheral nerves. The same lesions occur with the antihypertensive drug hydralazine (Raskin and Fishman, 1965). Malnutrition and vitamin B_6 deficiency favor development of neuropathy with both agents and prophylactic administration of the vitamin prevents it (Zbinden and Studer, 1955).

Other drugs which block pyridoxal phosphate include penicillamine and cycloserine. At sufficiently high doses bot agents may produce convulsions and cause a marked increase in xanthurenic acid excretion which is corrected with vitamin B_6 (Holtz and Palm, 1964). D-penicillamine, the isomer which should be used as drug of choice in man, is less toxic than L-penicillamine but can also cause biochemical signs of vitamin B_6 deficiency in rats (Asatoor, 1964) and man (Jaffe et al., 1964). Moreover, in one case of Wilson's disease development of optic axial neuritis was described after long-term treatment with the DL form of this drug. The clinical symptoms and the abnormal tryptophan loading test improved dramatically after the administration of large doses of vitamin B_6 (Tu et al., 1963). These examples demonstrate that blockade of pyridoxal phosphate by drugs may lead to a variety of clinical symptoms involving the central as well as the peripheral nervous system. One wonders and would like to speculate which other side-effects of the above-named drugs (and isoniazid, hydralazine, penicillamine, and cycloserine have many more!) might also be related to damage of a pyridoxal phosphate-containing enzyme. In rats at least, penicillamine also caused the typical vitamin B_6 deficiency symptom of the skin, acrodynia (Kuchinskas and duVigneaud, 1957). Such a change was never observed in my rats treated for short or long periods with isoniazid. This again shows that various drugs allegedly acting on the same biocatalyst and causing identical biochemical disturbances may produce quite different toxic lesions.

Recently, distinct changes in tryptophan metabolism have also been observed in many women taking oral contraceptives, suggesting a vitamin B_6 deficiency. Xanthurenic acid excretion, particularly after a tryptophan load, was markedly increased. It could be normalized by large doses of vitamin B_6 which also alleviated signs of depression in those unlucky subjects whose mood and sleep pattern steroid contraceptives had adversely affected (Luhby et al., 1971; Doberenz et al., 1971). The mechanism of the biochemical toxicity is not yet entirely clarified, although Rose and Braidman (1971) have submitted good arguments for an indirect action of the estrogens, i.e. a stimulation of tryptophan oxydase mediated via the hypothalamo-pituitary-adrenal axis.

IV

COMPARATIVE TOXICOLOGY

GENERAL REMARKS

The usefulness of animal experiments to predict drug toxicity in
man is not valued equally by all scientists engaged in evaluating the
potential risk of new chemicals. There are those who strongly believe
in the essential sameness of living organisms including man, this conviction culminating in such statements as "DNA is DNA". There are
others who, deep in their hearts, feel that animal experiments are a
waste of time and that only the crucial test in man will truly predict what a drug will do in man. These extreme views are so untenable
that they are rarely voiced in the open anymore. But one does not
have to be a toxicological radical to believe that species differences
constitute the most serious limiting factor in experimental drug toxicology. However, one should also not behave like a toxicological
chauvinist and use the species difference argument only to belittle a
harmful effect of one's drug; it matters just as much for negative
findings! Toxicological observations in animal model systems are to
be looked at as pieces of evidence, scientific facts which by themselves are neither good nor bad. To be fully understood, they must
be related to the clinical situation in which the drug will be used.
Comparative toxicology provides the necessary conversion tables which
help to put safety testing into proper perspective.

THE FACTOR AGE

That age of patients has something to do with frequency, severity and nature of toxic drug reactions every good doctor knows. It
is an equally accepted generalization that the age factor is particularly important for the very young and the very old. Toxicologists
have not kept aloof from this problem. The fact that they have
essentially contented themselves with the analysis of drug toxicity
in young animals is certainly due to the ease with which the appropriate test subjects can be procured. Moreover, toxic drug reactions
in the very young can often be explained by insufficiency of enzyme
systems, whereas in the old, a variety of degenerative processes and
diseases is thought to be responsible for many unusual drug effects.
However, this belief is not supported by many facts since few toxicologists have mustered the patience to obtain old animals and to do
the appropriate experiments.

How to Assess Drug Toxicity in Newborns and Infants

The immaturity of metabolic and excretory mechanisms and the incomplete development of tissues and organs make drug therapy of newborns and young infants a hazardous affair. The urgent need of pediatricians for toxicological information relevant for their excepttional patient population is therefore understandable. Faced with this pressing request and the huge number of drugs and other chemicals waiting to be tested, toxicologists tried to devise a convenient shortcut: they did LD_{50}'s in newborn rats and mice and compared them with those of mature animals. With official encouragement by regulatory agencies, innumerable litters of newborn mice and rats were sacrificed to this idea, and an enormous amount of toxicological data was accumulated (Goldenthal, 1971). Most of it is still waiting to be processed by comparative toxicology.

In short, the LD_{50} of certain drugs was found to be comparable in newborn and mature animals. With other compounds, however, it was considerably lower or considerably higher (Yeary et al., 1966). For example, the ratio of the s.c. LD_{50} in newborn and adult rats was about 1:1 for streptomycin sulfate, 1:2.5 for tetracycline HCl, 1:5 for erythromycin succinate, 1:7 for potassium penicillin G, 1:12.5 for lincomycin and 1:14 for chloramphenicol (Gray et al., 1966). In Goldenthal's (1971) tables of adult/newborn LD_{50} ratios, the highest is 750 for digoxin (p.o. rat), the lowest less than 0.02 for a vasoconstrictor amidephrine mesylate (p.o. rat). It is difficult to judge the practical value of this huge effort collectively undertaken by the toxicologists of the world. Some idea may perhaps be gained from a recently published experiment of Hudson et al. (1972). These authors determined the acute toxicity of 14 pesticides in ducks aged 1-1/2, 7, 30, and 180 days. Compared to adult birds young ducks were more sensitive to 6 and less sensitive to 8 compounds. At this point, it would be easy to insert a cheap joke, saying that such data were, of course, strictly for the birds. Doing this, I would again make the mistake of putting a value judgement on bits of scientific information. What these and similar experiments show is simply the fact that there are indeed important differences in toxicity of chemicals in young and adult animals and that such differences are most likely to exist also in man. What needs to be done is to find out the reasons for these differences. Once these are investigated, comparative toxicology must establish whether or not similar factors could operate in man.

Some of the factors which influence toxic effects of drugs in newborn and young animals can reasonably well be defined in terms of immaturity of specific enzyme activities, organ functions, and tissue differentiation. These are amenable to pharmacokinetic and pharmacodynamic analysis, and a direct comparison with the situation in human newborns and babies is often possible. Where such investigations fail to explain differences in susceptibility of young animals, a more imaginative vocabulary is needed to describe the observed phenomena. Differences in receptor responses, perhaps due to an incomplete inner organization of tissues and organs, different tissue composition, altered membrane permeability, and similar terms will have to be substituted for exact biochemical and physiological facts and figures. The following paragraphs will contain a few examples which illustrate various ways by which the toxicological role of the factor age may be assessed.

Pharmacokinetic Consideration

In evaluating the toxic potential of drugs for the newborn, the toxicologist is mainly concerned with those substances which exhibit unusually high acute toxicity in the LD_{50} screen. To explain such observations, a first possibility would be more rapid absorption of the drug from the gut or from injection sites. This mechanism was found to explain the high acute toxicity of 2 antihistamines, chlorpheniramine maleate and diphenhydramine, in very young rats (Lee, 1966). Antihistamines are also known to be poorly tolerated by young children and to cause occasionally severe convulsions. Thus, in this instance the animal test appears to have performed well, although the reason for the high incidence of toxic reactions in children has not yet been elucidated.

More often, toxic blood levels are a consequence of delayed drug excretion to which many factors contribute. First, take cognizance of the fact that the volume of extracellular fluid in the very young organism is about twice as large as in the adult. This physiological parameter can contribute towards delayed renal excretion. On the other hand, the intracellular fluid compartment is considerably smaller in the newborn than in the adult. Thus, drugs accumulating there are more likely to reach toxic levels (Burmeister, 1970). Another important and much more intensively investigated factor is the immaturity of drug metabolizing enzymes. In newborn rabbits, for example, such drugs as aminopyrine, amphetamine, acetanilide, chlorpromazine, and p-nitrobenzoic acid are not metabolized. At 2 weeks of age 5 to 37% of the enzyme activity is present and only after about 4 weeks are the adult levels of enzyme function reached (Fouts and Adamson, 1959). Similar observations were made in other laboratory animal species (Jondorf et al., 1959). One does not need much imagination to predict the deleterious effects should the above-mentioned and other lipid soluble drugs be given to the young and enzymatically unprepared test animals. The question then arises whether human newborns are any better able to detoxify such chemicals. Clinical studies indicate that they are not (Vest and Rossier, 1963). For example, a deficiency of enzymatic chloramphenicol conjugation was found to be responsible for an accumulation of the free antibiotic in the blood. When high doses were given to newborn babies, the drug caused severe, often lethal cardiovascular collapse, also known as "gray syndrome" (Lischner et al., 1961).

An interesting example of how differences in activity of drug metabolizing enzymes can help to solve a toxicological riddle was given by Allen and Chesney (1972). Their work pertains to the alkaloid monocrotaline which caused liver necrosis and pulmonary hypertension in small laboratory animals. In man and non-human primates, however, the striking pulmonary lesions did not occur. But when 4 week old monkeys were treated, typical pulmonary lesions with thickening and obliteration of arteries, leading to myocardial hypertrophy and right ventricular dilatation, developed. It could be explained by the inability of the young monkey's liver enzymes to produce the hepatotoxic metabolites of monocrotaline. Adult monkeys and human subjects accidentally exposed to the toxin apparently had a well-developed microsomal enzyme system and could convert the alkaloid readily to the hepatotoxic metabolites. Not answered as yet is the question of which other metabolite is responsible for the pulmonary lesions.

Increased drug toxicity in young animals can also be due to deficiencies in excretory mechanisms. It is established that tubular function of the kidney matures slowly not only in laboratory animals, but also in man (Dalton, 1970). An instructive example of how this can affect drug disposition was demonstrated with nalidixic acid in newborn and 7 month old calves by McChesney et al. (1969). Plasma half-life was 24 hrs in the newborn and traces of the drug were demonstrable for 15 days. In the older animals half-life was 90 minutes and complete clearance was rapid. The newborn calves were unable to concentrate the free drug in the urine and biliary excretion was high. 90 day old animals concentrated the drug in the urine 10 to 15 times compared to plasma values and excreted little with the bile. Drug metabolism in the adult human patient resembled that of the older calf, but the experiment in the human newborn which would make the comparative toxicologist happy, the authors unfortunately did not do.

A better penetration of drugs through biological membranes and into organs would constitute another mechanism by which toxic effects could be enhanced. For certain substances a better passage through the blood-brain barrier of young animals has been demonstrated (Ebert and Yim, 1961). An increase in permeability of the brain has also been established as the most likely cause of the high susceptibility of young rats to morphine (Kupferberg and Way, 1963). Of considerable practical importance is the blood-aqueous humor barrier which may not be well developed in young animals. High permeability could explain why 2,4-dinitrophenol caused lens opacities only in very young and not in older rabbits (Gehring and Buerge, 1969).

Unexplained Differences in Organ Sensitivity

Not unfrequently toxic drug effects are found to be either more or less severe or qualitatively different in young animals, although blood or tissue levels are not substantially different from those of the adult. This is particularly true for CNS-active drugs. As a general rule, newborns seem to be less sensitive to stimulants and more sensitive to depressants than mature animals (Yeary et al., 1966; Hudson et al., 1972). The depressant effect of pentobarbital shall be mentioned as an example. Its LD_{50} in newborn rats was about one third that of older animals. When drug concentrations were compared at lethal doses, the brain levels of the newborn were only about one third of those of adult rats, indicating a much higher sensitivity of the newborn's brain to the depressant effect of the barbiturate (Bianchine and Ferguson, 1967). That the opposite may also be true is shown by the example of diethylether. When rats were exposed to this drug at 15 or 20 Vol%, it took the very young 5 to 6 times longer to die than the adult animals. The blood levels of the drug measured at the time when 50% of the animals had died were up to 3 fold higher in the pups. Thus, not a reduced absorption of diethylether but an unexplained immaturity of the CNS must have protected the newborns (Schwetz and Becker, 1971). Qualitative differences in organ response to drugs are also occasionally found. For example, high doses of phenobarbital caused liver weight increase in young and old rats, but in young animals it was mostly due to cell proliferation, whereas in the adult rats, it was essentially a consequence of activated protein synthesis (Paulini et al., 1971). That toxic manifestations may also be qualitatively different is demonstrated by the example of calcium disodium edetate: treatment of very young rats caused liver necrosis; in 4 week old animals liver necrosis and mild kidney injury were seen, and in 12 week old rats the compound caused severe kidney lesions only (Reuber, 1967).

How then should we assess the toxic potential of drugs for newborns and babies? Certainly not by limiting our efforts to a comparison of LD50's in newborn and adult rats, although such experiments may have a certain value as a preliminary screening test. The examples have shown that metabolic differences must first be investigated; they are often responsible for an unusual reaction of the immature organism, and they can also be detected in human subjects. But in many instances, biochemical measurements will not explain differences in drug toxicity between newborns and adults. In such cases, it is, of course, easy to postulate a lag in tissue maturation, but it is difficult to obtain convincing evidence. Comparative embryological, histological, and histochemical studies are tedious and do not always solve the problems. That they may give important insight into the cause of toxic reactions is demonstrated by the work with monosodium glutamate, a compound which caused severe destructive lesions in the hypothalamus of newborn mice. This observation caused much concern, since the amino acid is also used to flavor baby food. Abraham et al. (1971) have carefully investigated the effect of monosodium glutamate and were able to relate it to a primary lesion of the lysosomes. But even with high doses, they were unable to produce brain damage in newborn monkeys. To explain this species difference, they recalled the fact that myelinization of the CNS in mice, rats, and rabbits starts 10 to 15 days after birth, which makes the 2-3 weeks after birth one of the vulnerable periods of the animals' CNS (Davison and Dobbing, 1966). In higher animals and man myelinization reaches its maximum before birth, and penetration of monosodium glutamate into the brain is therefore probably inhibited. This would explain the failure to induce brain lesions in newborn monkeys and would, at the same time, remove the concern that human babies might be injured by the compound.

Toxic Drug Reactions in Old Age

Ageing of tissues, decrease in enzyme activities, degenerative deterioration and higher incidence of diseases are factors thought to explain the higher susceptibility of old people for toxic drug reactions. Pharmacokinetic experiments can help to explain some of these differences. For example: meprobamate metabolism was found to be slower in old rats than in young animals, and it was noteworthy that stimulation by phenobarbital pretreatment was not very effective (Kato et al., 1961). Absorption and elimination of d-amphetamine injected s.c. into old rats were considerably delayed, brain levels were lower than in younger animals, but the pharmacologic response was more pronounced in the old rat. Moreover, on chronic treatment the old animals lost weight whereas younger rats given the same dose gained weight (Ziem et al., 1970). The experiment with d-amphetamine shows clearly that pharmacokinetic differences are only half of the story and that target organ response can also change with age. This was also demonstrated with ethanol, to which old rats were considerably more sensitive than young animals. In the old rats ethanol blood levels showed a slower decrease. In vitro, their livers metabolized the poison less rapidly, but biochemical studies showed that their livers contained considerably more alcohol dehydrogenase. The reason why the old rat's liver performed its duty less efficiently, is not known (Wiberg et al., 1970).

If ageing of tissues modifies drug effects, it is not surprising that this should be particularly conspicuous with reactions of the cardiovascular system. Clinical observations indicate that the regulatory mechanisms of blood pressure are upset more easily in the old patient. For example, i.v. injected propranolol caused greater decrease in systolic blood pressure in old subjects than in young volunteers (Conway, 1970). Severe orthostatic hypotension is a frequent and much feared side-effect of many drugs in the aged. It occurs particularly with neuroleptics, monoamine oxydase inhibitors, sympathetic and ganglionic blockers (Averbukh and Lapin, 1969). The myocardium becomes also more susceptible to injurious drug effects: Heart necroses induced by isoproterenol were more severe in old rats (Rona et al., 1959), focal myocardial degeneration after injection of pitressin were only seen in old but never in young cats (Dearing et al., 1944), and old dogs were more sensitive to acetylcholine-induced myocardial necroses (Hall et al., 1936). In man, digitalis toxicity is more prevalent in elderly patients (Soffer, 1961). This could be due to a higher sensitivity of the aged heart muscle, but there is also some evidence that enhanced toxicity is a consequence of impaired digitalis excretion (Chamberlain et al., 1970).

Sometimes drugs and degenerative diseases seem to function synergistically. This impression was gained from a study of various miotics administered locally for the purpose of treating glaucoma. During the clinical study the frequency of lens opacities increased in all patient groups, but the highest incidence of cortical lens alterations was found in the old age group treated with anticholinergic drugs (Abraham and Teller, 1969). It is obvious from these few examples that drug reactions in old age are dependent on a multiplicity of factors, many of them still poorly understood. There is no question that the old organism responds peculiarly to various exogenous stresses. This became evident when very old, mature, and young rats were subjected to various degrees of caloric malnutrition. Acute and subacute starvation which severely damaged young and mature animals did not seem to affect the old rats, their hemopoietic tissues were unchanged and their adrenals did not show signs of activation. But the picture changed when the old animals were subjected to chronic mild starvation: after varying time periods they suddenly showed severe signs of deterioration, indicating that their reserves and their regenerating ability were easily exhausted (Zbinden and Studer, 1956). These observations point to the need to study the ability of the old organism to repair the damage drugs very often do while they are performing their beneficial work. The tissues of young animals which we use in the conventional toxicity experiments have an extraordinary regenerating power. This vital force cannot be taken for granted in the old organism. Geriatric toxicology is therefore a subject which we can no longer afford to neglect.

AMBIENT TEMPERATURE

An extensive literature has accumulated on the modification of drug effects by ambient temperature (Fuhrman and Fuhrman, 1961; Weihe, 1973). Toxicologists have contributed much to it. Unfortunately, most investigators contented themselves with measurements of LD_{50}'s of mice and rats at various temperatures, as if death were not only the most conveniently determined but also the most relevant endpoint in drug toxicology.

From these studies we are well informed now that acute toxicity of some drugs, particularly those which stimulate heat production, shows a linear relationship to ambient temperature. This effect, most prominently demonstrated with sympathomimetic amines, is even more pronounced in crowded animals where heat dissipation is impaired and discomfort is multiplied by displeasing company. With many other drugs acute toxicity increases both above and below a certain temperature somewhere between room temperature and thermal neutrality. Thus, if toxicity is plotted against ambient temperature, a U-shaped curve is found. The group of compounds behaving in this manner includes many which affect the CNS, such as phenothiazines, monoamine oxidase inhibitors, reserpine, and salicylates. There may be a third type of drugs whose toxicity only increases above the thermoneutral zone, but remains unchanged at lower temperatures. Procaine and caffeine can be mentioned as examples (Fuhrman and Fuhrman, 1961).

Do these studies have any relevance for man? Apart from such unreasonable exercises as swimming in an ice-cold lake at Christmas or sitting naked in the infernal heat of a Finnish sauna or, worst of all, doing the former after the latter, civilized man rarely exposes himself unprotected to extreme temperatures. And in contrast to small laboratory animals, we not only combat overheating with sweat but have learned to maintain a comfortable climate under our clothing and bed sheets. Thus, variations of our ambient temperature are not of such magnitude that they would constitute an important factor in human responses to drugs. An exception are those compounds which interfere with thermoregulation, particularly perspiration. It is an often quoted fact that discomfort from atropin is greatly increased in patients living in hot and humid environments. But it is less well known that treatment with phenothiazines can induce hyperthermia during heat spells. Weihe (1973) has discovered several cases described in the psychiatric literature coming from such hot spots as Waco, Texas; Topeka, Kansas; and New York City.

A somewhat different problem is that of changed responsiveness to drugs after prolonged exposure to extreme ambient temperatures. In small animals, acclimatization to low temperature causes an overall increase in body metabolism (Depocas et al., 1957). In rats this was coupled with a 1,000 to 10,000 fold higher sensitivity to the toxic action of isoproterenol (Balazs et al., 1962). But toxicity of other drugs is decreased in cold-adapted animals, an example being atropin. In this case, not an increase in metabolic rate but a delayed absorption from i.p. injection site was found to be the explanation of the lower toxicity (Kalser et al., 1967). Moreover, cold adaptation also increased protein binding of the drug.

In conclusion, comparative toxicology has uncovered so many differences in the adaptive processes to extreme temperatures between small laboratory animals and man that the interesting relationships between ambient temperature and LD_{50} seem to be of little relevance for human drug therapy. Those drugs which affect our temperature regulation, however, are potentially dangerous even at ambient temperatures common to places where many people live. Acclimatization to extreme temperatures causes important metabolic changes whose significance as contributing factor to drug toxicity needs to be investigated further.

V

PHARMACODYNAMIC TOXICOLOGY

GENERAL REMARKS

Pharmacodynamics is the science which studies the biochemical and physiological effects of drugs and attempts to explain their mechanism of action. Pharmacodynamic toxicology does exactly the same thing but must keep its hands off the therapeutically useful actions and be content with the undesired ones. No one will deny that it is a much neglected branch of toxicology, and always has been. Geoffrey Woodard knew it when he wrote almost 20 years ago: "All too often in the pressure of events involved in obtaining data to support the safety of a chemical for use by man, the pharmacodynamic study is relegated to second place or forgotten entirely. In other cases, the pharmacodynamic study came as an afterthought when it became apparent that certain observations made during the course of the classical toxicity studies needed explanation." (Lehman et al., 1955)

Pharmacologists have been suspected of subconsciously neglecting to investigate the undesired properties of their drugs, just like a parent who prefers not to know about undesired activities of his off-spring. The reluctance to lend their skills for toxicological studies may also be explained by the fact that many pharmacological test methods are just not adaptable to yield relevant safety information (Zbinden, 1966b). Moreover, some people still equate functional toxi-city--the kind pharmacodynamic studies might detect--with reversible and therefore harmless side-effects. But functional drug reactions are not always reversible and certainly not always harmless. Regard-less of the "pressure of events" pharmacodynamic studies must be in-corporated into the preclinical evaluation of a new drug.

Probably more important than a somewhat dull screening for all kinds of potential functional side-effects is the use of pharmacody-namics when "certain observations made during the course of the classical toxicity studies need explanations." Since the toxicologist by tradition, by law, and by regulations, must induce a maximum of damaging effects in his experiments, he needs all help he can get in-cluding that of pharmacodynamics to explain the harm done to the ani-mals and to provide convincing arguments why the drug may still be given to patients.

THYROID STIMULATION

Anybody doing routinely chronic toxicity studies with drugs or pesticides will sooner or later come across a compound which inter-

feres with organic binding of iodine in the thyroid, causes enlargement of the gland, and is therefore classified as a goitrogen.
Histologically, the thyroids of these animals show a pretty picture
with characteristic high columnar epithelial cells which almost obli-
terate the lumen of the follicles. The colloid is pale staining,
often missing, and capillaries are abundant.

Already in 1943 Astwood was able to list some 40 goitrogens
which could be grouped chemically into (1) thiourea and related compounds, e.g., thiouracil, 2-thiobarbituric acid, and thiosemicarba-
zide, (2) certain aniline derivatives, e.g., sulfonamides and p-aminobenzoic acid, and (3) cyanides and thiocyanates. Many others were
added since, e.g., aminotriazole (Fregly, 1968), a herbicide about
which toxicologists like to make a few jokes on Thanksgiving Days,
long acting sulfonamides (Randall et al., 1959), chlorpropamide and
an antifertility compound U 11634 (5-(α,α,α-trifluoro-tolyloxymethyl)-
2-oxazolidinethione (Webster et al., 1967).

If such compounds are fed to laboratory animals at high doses
for a year or more, multiple adenomas may develop in the hyperplastic
thyroid gland. Later, the thyroid tissue often invades blood vessels
which are always abundant and engorged. Sometimes metastases of the
thyroid tissue are disseminated into the lungs and only the lungs.
Pharmacodynamic toxicology has gone at great length to explain this
unusual observation. It has established that the development of thyroid tumors in goitrogen-treated animals is due to hypersecretion of
thyroid stimulating hormone (TSH) by the anterior lobe of the pitui-
tary gland. To remove even the slightest doubt that not only the
thyroid hyperplasia but also the induction of metastasizing tumors
(called thyroid carcinomas by many pathologists) were all the doings
of TSH and not perhaps related to a hidden carcinogenic effect of the
drugs themselves, a number of ingenious experiments were devised.
They showed that thyroid hyperplasia and tumor formation did not occur
in goitrogen-treated mice and rats which received small shots of thy-
roxin or whose TSH secretion was cut off by hypophysectomy (Astwood,
1943). The process could even be interrupted at a higher level, i.e.,
by an experimental lesion of the anterior hypothalamus (Kavetsky et
al., 1969). The quite unusual ability of thyroid tissue to settle in
the lungs was extensively studied by Taptiklis (1968, 1969). He
injected thyroid cells from normal, hyperplastic, and tumorous glands
of mice into untreated and goitrogen-treated mice. The cells failed
to take in normal mice but grew rapidly in the lungs and in no other
tissue of recipients whose thyroid function was suppressed by methyl-
thiouracil. Thyroid growth in the lungs also occurred in animals
treated with I^{131}. The strange relationship between thyroid and lung
is further illustrated by Taptiklis' observation that i.v. injected
thyroid cells appeared to lay dormant in the lungs of normal mice for
many months. They started to grow and to form detectable lung metastases only after thyroid function was suppressed.

These pharmacodynamic studies have helped to weigh the risk of
goitrogens for man by proving that thyroid hyperplasia and tumor formation only occur if drugs are given at doses which inhibit thyroid
function, a parameter which is readily measured in man. Sulfonamides,
for example, act as goitrogens in rats and dogs where they suppress
thyroid function. Man and monkey, however, are less sensitive and do
not even show a hint of impaired thyroid function when treated with
the customary therapeutic doses. Pharmacodynamic toxicology can

therefore predict with confidence that these drugs will not be goitro-
genic in man and do not constitute a carcinogenic hazard for man
either.

The situation is different with thiouracil and related compounds
which are given for the express purpose of inhibiting thyroid function. Man responds to these compounds with hyperplasia of thyroid
tissue, deformation of follicles with papillary growth, and sometimes
signs of malignant degeneration (Hedinger and Egloff, 1967). At this
point pharmacodynamic toxicology ends. It cannot tell us whether
metastatic spread may happen in man after prolonged treatment with
thyreostatic drugs. Pathologists feel that it is not likely to occur.
This impression is confirmed by Nature's own experiment, the rare
cases of congenital impairment of thyroid hormone synthesis. In these
patients there is an impressive enlargement of the thyroid often with
atypical proliferation of the glandular tissue but without metastatic
propagation (Vilde and Nezelof, 1966; Hedinger and Egloff, 1967).

VI

SYMPTOMATIC TOXICOLOGY

GENERAL REMARKS

What the detective novel is to fiction, symptomatic toxicology is to clinical therapeutics. Its stories are about bad deeds, committed not by a criminal, but by a drug. All the elements of an Agatha Christie thriller are there: A person is harmed and a number of drugs are immediately suspected as perpetrators; but there are few clues on which to convict the culprit. The toxicological detective must laboriously put together his circumstantial evidence, and quite often he must wait until the villain strikes again and again. Then too, many of the suspects have excellent advocates and friends in high places; they are important members of the therapeutic armamentarium, benefactors of society and may have saved the life of many of our fellow citizens. Truly, to watch these great cases of symptomatic toxicology unfold from the first suspicion voiced in a letter to the editor of Lancet to the public tribunal to which experts of all vocations contribute is much more interesting than to watch masked men holding up a bank. Many books are written and motion pictures are made about cops and robbers, but the intricate stories of highly promising drugs with their fatal attributes, their bad deeds, their prosecution, and their ultimate conviction are rarely told.

But as life in court does not only consist of capital crimes, symptomatic toxicology must also deal with many petty offenses. Just about every vital function and biochemical reaction may be adversely affected by drugs. Although this is quite often of little significance and may be acceptable to the doctor and even to the patient as a price to pay for the drug's beneficial effect, symptomatic toxicology must recognize and register every compound's imperfections. The complicity of drugs in the development of many derangements of organ functions must be exposed pitilessly. It should not be done, however, as a pretext to discourage the use of chemotherapeutic agents but as an auxiliary means for their better deployment.

OXALURIA

Historical Reminiscence

It may be appropriate to use as a first example of the Chapter on Symptomatic Toxicology a classical case which has greatly affected development of drug toxicology. In 1937 a small amount, exactly 11 gallons and 6 pints, of a sufanilamide elixir was dispensed on the American market. The drug contained 72% diethylene glycol as solvent a substance which was soon found to be highly nephrotoxic. Half of the above-named amount was consumed. As a consequence, more than 100 people died within days. This tragic accident not only started an exemplary toxicological emergency operation but was also the immediate inducement for a comprehensive revision and tightening of the U S Food, Drug and Cosmetic Act (Geiling and Cannon, 1938). After this safety testing of drugs became a rigidly regulated and controlled procedure.

In the course of the experimental evaluation of diethylene glycol and related compounds, it became clear that this class of chemicals possessed unusual nephrotoxic properties. Several analogs also caused hyperoxaluria with precipitation of Ca oxalate crystals in the kidney and stone formation (Doerr et al., 1947). Particularly useful for this experimental model was ethylene glycol, a substance which also became a toxicological problem itself, since it was widely distributed as antifreeze. There seems to be no practicable way to prevent people from keeping it in Burgundy bottles and to drink it accidentally. Thus, we are constantly reminded that chemicals can affect oxalic acid excretion and that this may be dangerous to their health.

Metabolic Data

The key intermediate in oxalate metabolism is glyoxylate which is formed from various sources, e.g., glycine, glycolate and, of course, ethylene glycol. It may be converted by several enzymes to oxalate, but competitively it is also transaminated to glycine (Richardson, 1967). In man normal daily oxalate excretion is not more than 40 mg (Hodgkinson and Zarembski, 1968). In primary hyperoxaluria, an inherited disease which is due to a deficiency of the enzyme catalyzing transamination of glyoxylate to glycine, oxalate excretion is increased to 100-400 mg per 24 hrs or more. The major symptoms are nephrolithiasis and severe kidney blockade. A similar metabolic defect may be acquired by vitamin B_6 deficiency which is associated with hyperoxaluria in animals as well as in man (Wyngaarden and Elder, 1966).

If you want to demonstrate precipitation of oxalate crystals in kidneys of rats, you can administer 0.25% of ethylene glycol or more in their drinking water. But you better use male animals which perform more reliably than females in this experiment. This is probably due to the fact that testosterone activates glycolic acid oxydase and increases glyoxylate and oxalate production (Richardson, 1967). Oxalate excretion is also increased in animals on high purine diet and by vitamin D and estrogen, the latter two agents acting probably via an effect on calcium metabolism (Hodgkinson and Zarembski, 1968).

Toxicological Implications

That accidental ingestion of oxalic acid and poisonous oxalate precursors can cause kidney damage which is at least partly due to precipitation of Ca oxalate was mentioned above. The question now is, could certain drugs act in a similar fashion and facilitate kidney stone formation through an effect on oxalate metabolism? To

evaluate this question, some clinical facts regarding the relations-
ship between oxalate metabolism and nephrolithiasis must be considered.

The majority of kidney stones occurring in Western populations
contain oxalates (Zarembski and Hodgkinson, 1969). Most probably the
stones are formed from small aggregates of Ca oxalate crystals (Dyer
and Nordin, 1967). The formation of Ca oxalate concrements depends
on the solubility product of Ca and oxalate ions in the urine (v.
Sengbusch and Sücker, 1966). It is somewhat disquieting to know that
even in normal urines Ca oxalate is often present in a super-satura-
ted solution, to be exact, in 44% of all day portions and 71% of the
night urines (Elliot and Ribeiro, 1967). There are, fortunately,
substances in the urine such as glucuronides, inorganic pyrophosphate
and urinary peptides, which function as solubilizers and prevent precipitation of oxalate microcrystals (Hodgkinson and Zarembski, 1968).

Kidney stones can therefore develop through three mechanisms:
(1) excessive oxalate excretion, (2) breakdown of the solubilizing
power of the urine, and (3) increased aggregation of microcrystals.
About 80% of patients suffering from oxalate-containing kidney stones
excrete less than 15 mg oxalate per day (Desgrez et al., 1968). This
means that the second and third mechanisms, together with anatomical
abnormalities in the urinary system, must be of foremost etiological
importance. This does not prove that oxalate excretion is irrelevant.
On the contrary, in nephrolithiasis patients showing high oxalate
excretion, the disease usually takes a more progressive course.
(Desgrez et al., 1968) Thus, the advice of doctors to their nephrolithiasis patients to avoid spinach, rhubarb, and similar delicacies
remains a sound prophylactic measure (v.Sengbusch and Timmermann,
1957).

In evaluating drugs as contributing factors in kidney stone formation, first those which increase oxalic acid excretion should be
mentioned. Of these ascorbic acid has attracted some attention recently due to L. Pauling's recommendation to use this vitamin in
daily doses up to 15 g to prevent and treat common cold. Since 40-
50% of the oxalates normally present in urine are derived from the
ascorbic acid of the food (Baker et al., 1962; Atkins et al., 1965),
the possibility that such large amounts of vitamin C could lead to
hyperoxaluria should at least be considered. All those believing in
the curative power of ascorbic acid can be reassured that our body
has neither the intention nor enough enzymes to metabolize large quantities of their wonderdrug. Up to about 3 g per day (which should be
all anybody would want to take) no significant increase in oxalate
excretion was found. However, a moderate but significant increase in
urinary oxalates was demonstrated after daily intake of 4 g, and after
9 g, oxalate excretion increased an average of 68 mg above base values
with a maximum increase in some volunteers of 150 mg per 24 hrs (Lamden and Chrystowski, 1954). This, of course, are amounts seen in
primary hyperoxaluria. I cannot believe that prolonged iatrogenic
hyperoxaluria of such magnitude should be a perfectly harmless or even
recommendable metabolic deviation.

Other drugs which increase oxalate excretion are those which
cause vitamin B_6 deficiency by forming a complex with pyridoxal phosphate (see page 36). This vitamin functions as a coenzyme of the
enzyme which converts glyoxylate to glycine. If it is blocked more
oxalic acid is formed. The important example is isoniazid which caused

hyperoxaluria in rats, particularly in those which were kept on a pyridoxine-free diet (Gershoff and Faragalla, 1959). Isoniazid also causes disturbance of vitamin B_6 metabolism in man and could therefore also increase oxalate excretion, particularly in poorly nourishe tuberculous patients.

The two other factors in kidney stone formation, reduction of the solubilizing power of urine and facilitation of aggregate formation of microcrystals, are much more difficult to assess. Von Sengbusch and Timmermann (1957) have developed a method which permits counting of microcrystals of 60 μ diameter and more in the urine. To do it one needs a special sieve and a dedicated technician. With this method it could be shown that even in normals the number of micro stones increased significantly after administration of oxalate-rich food. The same happened after intake of a single dose of 6 g ascorbic acid. It is suggested (but far from proved) that this method can assess the tendency of oxalate microcrystals to form microstones, some of which could, under favorable conditions, develop into kidney stones

Toxicologists have made limited efforts to find an experimental approach to the problem. The model they are using to study drug effects on kidney stone formation consists of implanting lead globules or small glass pearls in the bladder of experimental animals. After an appropriate time during which part of the animals are subjected to drug treatment, the foreign bodies on which salts have precipitated are removed. Concrement formation is measured by weight increase of the foreign bodies and chemical analysis of the precipitates. Ascorbic acid has been tested in this system using lead globules implanted into the bladders of rats. Compared to controls, it caused a higher weight increase of the precipitates which was due to deposition of oxalates (Takenouchi et al., 1966). Such experiments must be looked at as preliminary screens, simplified models for the very intricate process of kidney stone formation. On the other hand, they introduce the factor of local inflammation and irritation which may be very important in many cases of nephrolithiasis.

In summary, a number of drugs have been found to increase oxalate excretion in the urine by various biochemical mechanisms. The significance of this biochemical effect for kidney stone formation in man remains to be established.

ACUTE, INTERSTITIAL, EOSINOPHILIC MYOCARDITIS

Symptoms and Pathology

Allergic skin reactions to serums, vaccines and drugs are occasionally accompanied by signs of cardiovascular injury ranging from mild dyspnea and precordial pain to acute cor pulmonale, cardiac failure and even myocardial infarct. In the ECG various changes of the T wave and the ST segment may, but must not, be present. All changes usually disappear within a few days. In rare cases cardiac failure and shock developed, and the patients succumbed to what first seemed to be a trite annoyance (Bickel, 1960).

In the few lethal cases who came to autopsy, an impressive acute diffuse interstitial myocarditis was found. There were extensive

focal destructions of myocardial fibers, marked proliferation of the
connective tissue, occasionally forming tuberculoid granulomas, and
an almost unbelievable accumulation of eosinophilic leukocytes accompanied by Charcot-Leyden crystals. In some cases numerous myoge-
nic and mesenchymal giant cells were seen. Blood vessels were usually spared, although there were cases with a necrotizing inflammation
of small arteries (Klinge, 1966; Schwartz, 1968; Batzenschlager et al,
1970; and personal observation). In one case of allergic myocarditis
due to aminosalicylic acid, IgG could be demonstrated in the areas of
myocardial necrosis by immunofluorescent technique (Barrett et al,
1971).

Experimental Equivalents and Offending Drugs

Myocarditis occurring with drug-induced skin reactions is thought
to be an allergy comparable to lesions induced experimentally by repeated injections of foreign proteins. When anaphylactic shock was
induced in rabbits by injection of horse serum, ECG changes of various
kinds were found and could be explained by allergic myocarditis seen
histopathologically. In these animals, vascular changes such as fi-
brinoid necrosis of the media of arteries with lymphoplasmocellular
infiltrations was always present. It was also quite interesting to
note that ECG changes developed in all sensitized and rechallenged
animals including those which did not experience any visible signs of
shock (Bickel, 1960). With small molecules, e.g. drugs, these injuries cannot be produced in animals.

To no one's surprise, neoarsphenamine was the first substance to
cause allergic myocarditis. Since then several drugs known to cause
frequent skin eruptions in man have also been associated with a case
or two of eosinophilic myocarditis. This includes aspirin and various
analgesic mixtures, phenindione, penicillin, sulfonamides, colimycin,
carbamazepine, and an unspecified iodine-preparation (Zeh and Klaus,
1962; Schröpl and Stollmann, 1967; Schwartz, 1968:, Batzenschlager et
al, 1970). These are, as mentioned single cases, examples of what
appears to be a very rare disease. Considering the fact that skin
reactions to drugs are by far the most frequent morphologically demonstrable drug reaction, it seems somewhat strange that concomitant
myocarditis should be so rare. In its mild form it might be much
more frequent, however. This can be derived from the interesting results of Bickel's effort who carefully monitored the ECG of patients
with drug-induced skin eruptions. He reported ECG changes such as
troubles of conductivity, excitability and coronary flow in many cases
of drug allergies, chiefly those with skin symptoms. These were particularly frequent after treatment with serums, vaccines, sulfonamides
and penicillin. Changes of the T-wave after allergic reaction to
penicillin were also present in three patients of Binder et al (1950).
They experienced no subjective cardiovascular symptoms and recovered
in a few days (Binder et al, 1950). It is probable that such patients
had mild disseminated myocardial fiber necrosis, a lesion which cannot
be fully reversible, but would leave tiny scars scattered throughout
the heart muscle. If this were the case, allergic skin reactions to
drugs could never be regarded as an insignificant accompaniment of
drug therapy but should be accepted as a serious complication to be
avoided whenever possible. Having seen a patient die from eosinophilic myocarditis after being rechallenged with the purpose of identify-
ing the suspected allergen, I cannot but feel that this cautious attitude has some justification.

COOMBS TEST POSITIVITY

Drug Toxicity as a Scientific Bonus

Each drug administration to a human subject is in itself a small experiment in clinical pharmacology. The therapeutic effect is considered the regular pay-off, the undesired side-reaction the price to pay for the benefit. But sometimes an unexpected bonus accrues from unpleasant drug toxicity, in that it opens up new approaches to the study of biological functions and the understanding of pathological processes. What would cell physiology be without the knowledge gained from the toxic effects of anticancer drugs? Didn't neurophysiology profit from clinical observations of undesired effects of compounds depleting or increasing brain amines? Haven't the many side-effects of cortisone shed new light on mineral, fat and carbohydrate metabolism, blood pressure regulation and the function of lymphocytes? These examples show that drugs have become invaluable research tools. This is an important contribution of pharmaceutical research which has never really been adequately acknowledged and appreciated.

Drugs Behind a Positive Direct Coombs Test

Many patients, perhaps 20%, taking α-methyldopa for several months develop a positive direct Coombs antiglobulin test. It detects antibodies of the pure gamma G type having some rhesus specificity. They are self-sufficient, i.e., they act in the test tube with the patient's own red cells in the absence of drug or metabolites. Symptoms of hemolytic anemia such as reticulocytosis, spherocytosis, bilirubinemia, shortened erythrocyte survival and splenomegaly are found only in a small percentage of the cases. (Carstairs et al, 196 Worlledge et al, 1966; LoBuglio and Jandl, 1967). The immunological mechanism has not yet been fully elucidated, but many unique features have been brought to the open (Worlledge et al, 1966). Recently a similar effect was observed with mefenamic acid which caused autoimmune hemolytic anemia in 3 patients and a positive direct Coombs test without anemia in 1 out of 36 subjects taking the drug for 3 or more months. As in most patients on α-methyldopa, the Coombs test remained positive for several months after discontinuation of therapy (Scott et al., 1968).

The mode of action of α-methyldopa is, as mentioned, not yet fully understood, but its mechanism can be distinguished from other forms of drug-induced Coombs test positivity. One of these goes under the name of "innocent bystander mechanism". Here, antibodies are directed against the drug. The drug-antibody complexes attach to the innocent bystanders, the red cells, thereby splashing them with complement protein. Thus, the direct Coombs test is positive with anti-complement, but not with anti-gamma G serum. Hemolysis or premature destruction of the complement-coated red cells in the reticuloendothelial system may ensue. Drugs associated with this type of reaction are stibophen, quinine, quinidine, phenacetin, and Sedormid[R] (Croft et al., 1968). The latter compound is still remembered for its association with thrombocytopenia which shows that sometimes, for unknown reasons, the immunological misfortune may hit another bystander.

A rare form of drug-induced Coombs test positive hemolytic anemia may occur after large doses of penicillin. Gamma G antibodies are present in the serum and on the surface of red cells. But the serum antibodies hemolyze normal erythrocytes only in the presence of the drug, suggesting a hapten-type mechanism (Croft et al., 1968).

A positive direct Coombs test develops also in up to 75% of patients taking the antibiotic cephalothin; the reaction is apparently due to a non-specific coating of red cells with a cephalothin-globulin complex and has, therefore, no immunological basis. The test was found positive particularly in azotemic patients. This was due to higher drug blood levels, reduced protein binding owing to low albumin levels and a higher tendency of the red cells to aggregate. The reaction must be considered more as a laboratory curiosity and could not be related to an autoimmune hemolytic state (Molthan et al., 1967; Gralnick et al., 1967). With the closely related cephalosporin antibiotic, cephaloridine, the incidence of positive direct Coombs test was only 8%. Positivity was most frequent in patients with long-term and high-dose treatment (Fass et al., 1970).

VII

SYSTEMATIC TOXICOLOGY

GENERAL REMARKS

On their daily rounds clinicians are often confronted with new symptoms suggesting an unexpected evolution of their patients' ailments. An adverse drug effect is one of many causes of such disturbing developments. The knowledge that similar symptoms have been induced in animals by a drug the patient is taking or were observed in equally treated patients before, reinforces the suspicion that a toxic reaction may have taken place. On the other hand, if the effect has never been linked to drug therapy in animals or man, the question of a toxic reaction will figure much less prominently in the clinician's differential dignostic considerations.

We all would like to have a computer terminal in our offices in which to feed the names of all drugs a patient has taken together with the code of the new symptoms giving us diagnostic problems. The computer would then search its memory and print the probability that the reaction was due to a toxic effect for each drug and drug combination Lacking such a service, clinicians must consult package inserts which contain little toxicological data but often an almost endless list of side-effects uncritically compiled from clinical observations. What is usually lacking is an up-to-date registry of selected toxicologica. data with some informed discussion of its significance for the drug's use in man. Just how useful such background information can be shall be explored in the following examples.

HEXACHLOROPHENE

Problems of Communication

Recent experience with hexachlorophene (HCP) has again demonstrated how difficult it sometimes is to obtain systematic toxicological background data and how important such information can become under certain circumstances. As it was pointed out earlier, routine toxicological testing assures the physician that the drug has undergone a certain minimum of experimental investigations, that a substantial number of animals has been treated with sufficiently high doses, that blood, urine, and organ functions were checked and that most organs were examined histologically. This information, despite its shortcomings, can be used as a point of reference from which to start more sophisticated investigations should the experimental or the later clinical observations point to a need for further studies. For vari-

ous reasons these data are, however, rarely published and remain
locked away in the files of drug companies and government agencies.
Moreover, they are not regularly updated as the state of the art in
toxicology develops, a fact which becomes painfully obvious for any-
one who reviews the toxicological background data of many of our
older and still widely used drugs, not to speak of many food additives
which have been around for years.

Systematic Toxicology of HCP

HCP is a disinfectant which was introduced in 1945 as an addi-
tive to soap. It later became an increasingly popular ingredient of
many toiletry products. A review of its toxicological properties
published in 1969 by Gump illustrates the problems alluded to above;
as to completeness of data: the review clearly reflects the state of
the art of the early days of toxicology. For example, the only subacute study is an economy model, an experiment in which groups of 6
rats were treated with 0.02 and 0.04% HCP as admixture to the diet
for 30 days. As to the availability of the data, many of the routine
toxicity tests mentioned in Gump's (1969) review were done by private
laboratories and not published. The one subacute oral test mentioned
above is summarized in two sentences from which only a fraction of
the intrinsic informational value of the experiment can be gained.
Having lived through the past 20 years of toxicological progress, I
am the last to criticize the work of our predecessors. In my view
Gump should be commended for having made background information on
HCP toxicology available to the scientific community. His review
represents a very instructive case on which one can demonstrate how
scientific progress may call in doubt long established beliefs.

The second chapter of the story of HCP toxicology began when
manufacturers expressed the desire to expand the compound's use as a
fungicide for various foodstuffs (Lockhart, 1972). This prompted two
scientists of the Food and Drug Administration to conduct new subacute toxicity studies in rats. Using modern methods of neuropathology, they were surprised to find an ususual toxic effect, cerebral
edema affecting exclusively the white matter of the brain and spinal
cord, a spongiform encephalopathy which transformed the white matter
into an almost unbelievable network of cystic spaces lined by frag-
ments of myelin (Kimbrough and Gaines, 1971). Electron microscopic
studies demonstrated degeneration of myelin. Nerve cells appeared to
be unchanged, and the lesions were shown to be reversible, although
it took many weeks for all the holes in the white matter to disappear.

It is quite in order that toxicological data of older drugs are
reevaluated whenever the compound's field of indications is widened,
when its worldwide sales show a substantial and steady increase or
when the substance is recommended in higher doses and for longer
periods of time. Such reevaluations may often indicate the need for
additional animal tests even with compounds which are GRAS (generally
recognized as safe). As in the case of HCP, these studies may un-
earth hitherto unrecognized toxic effects, and thereby present manufacturers and health authorities with a difficult problem. The
situation is often critical because the substance may already be in
everybody's medicine cabinet or in every girl's underarm deodorant,
and a regulatory action must be taken long before a thorough scientific evaluation has been completed. What is needed in such cases is

a prompt realization of the missing toxicological experiments, an action which is presently underway in what may be called the 3rd phase of HCP systematic toxicology. Although only a few studies have been published, it is confirmed that the main target organ for HCP toxicity is the white matter of the central nervous system. The drug seems to act on mitochondrial metabolism (Cammer and Moore, 1972) which may be the primary lesion leading to myelin degeneration. We have also found mild focal degeneration of peripheral nerves in rats characterized by grotesque ballooning of myelin sheath followed by destruction (Zbinden and Alder, 1973). In animal experiments there seems to be a good relationship between dose, blood levels, morphological and functional disturbances of the nervous system (Lockhart, 1972). No unusual species differences have so far been detected. Good absorption through unbroken, and particularly also burned skin was demonstrated. Correlations between blood levels and histological findings in animals are summarized in Table 10, together with blood level data obtained in man. From this collection it is clear that HCP is readily absorbed through the human skin but does not accumulate appreciably in the body. Its safety margin appears to be narrow. It follows that misuse, be it through oral ingestion of HCP-containing lotions or overuse on the skin, for example, in the treatment of burns, can lead to acute poisoning. Several such cases have occurred and were reviewed by Kimbrough (1971) and Lockhart (1972). The leading symptoms reflect the neurotoxic properties of the compound and include coma, spasms, convulsions, nausea, and vomiting. A tragic confirmation of the narrowness of HCP's safety margin occurred recently in France where hundreds of babies became ill and over 30 died after being treated with powder containing the excessive amount of 5% of the disinfectant (Pines, 1972). This, of course, would not have happened with the correct formulation. But, we may ask, were the basic facts of HCP's systematic toxicology known to the people responsible for manufacturing the deadly baby powder and to those involved in selling countless other products containing this compound? Or were they perhaps overconfident that good old HCP that had been around for over 30 years was harmless? Were they aware of the dramatic encephalopathy this compound can cause in animals and probably also in man? Did they have ready access to these basic toxicological facts? The answers to these questions are not known. But since there are many other widely used chemicals whose toxicology is also not common knowledge, I doubt that chemists and pharmacists were aware of the toxicological background of HCP. Even if they had the facts and figures, how many were trained in toxicology enough to be able to judge the human risk involved in its use?

Should the use of HCP be regulated and how? The various countries have taken different actions: The U S Food and Drug Administration permits the compound only in prescription products except in very low concentrations as a preservative. The IKS, The Swiss regulatory body, has banned it from baby powders and requires a warning statement on products containing 3% HCP not to use them for whole body washings of babies and on burned skin. My own feeling is that HCP should be used as a disinfectant in effective concentrations, in the operating room and in the general hospital practice. But there is no need to build up unnecessary blood and tissue levels in the population at large through continuous exposure to low, not very effective and certainly not necessary concentrations in toiletry products. A similar recommendation comes from Plueckhahn and Banks (1972) who base their judgement of HCP's safety and usefulness on many years of experience in over 25,000 babies.

TABLE 10

Blood Levels and Toxic Effects of HCP in Animals and Man

Species	Dose and Method of Application	Time Days	Blood Levels ug/ml Mean	Minimal	Maximal	Encepha- lopathy	Ref.
Man/ Newborn	(Cord blood)	−	0.022	0.003	0.082	−	1
Man/ Newborn	Daily wash, 3% prep. diluted	1-11	0.109	−	0.646	−	1
Man/ Newborn	Daily wash, 3% prep.	1-5	0.34	−	−	−	2
Man/Pre- mature	Daily wash, 3% prep.	24	1.1*	−	−	−	2
Man	5 daily handwashings, 1 min., 3% prep.	28	0.07	−	−	−	2
Man	3 daily hand and face wash- ings, 3% prep.	28	0.196	−	−	−	2
Man	5 daily surgical scrubs of hands, 10 min., 3% prep.	10	−	−	0.1	−	2
Man	2 daily body washings, 3% soap	60	0.68	0.25	1.08	−	2
Monkey/ Newborn	Daily washings, 3% prep.	90	1.1- 1.5	−	−	+	2
rat	20 ppm p.o.	258	0.28	0.198	0.324	0	2
rat	100 ppm p.o.	258	1.21	−	−	+	2
rat	200 ppm p.o.	84	−	0.4	0.8	0	2
rat	500 ppm p.o.	98	−	−	−	+	3
rat	2x 5 mg/kg p.o. 5 times per week	35	−	−	−	0	4
rat	2x 10 or 2x 15 mg/kg p.o. 5 times per week	5-35	−	−	−	+	4

Ref.: 1: Curley et al. 1971, 2: Lockhart 1972, 3: Kimbrough and Gaines 1971,
       4: Alder and Zbinden (unpublished)

− not known
0 not present
+ present
* one individual only

HYPERVITAMINOSIS

A Problem to be Concerned about?

In the preceding section I listed various reasons which would compel one to review and perhaps amend toxicological background data of widely distributed, long established and apparently safe drugs. Among them were: A steady and substantial increase in sales of a certain compound, evidence that it is prescribed either for additional diseases, at substantially higher doses or for longer periods of time, and, I may add, if there is widespread overuse without effective medical supervision.

Vitamins certainly are long established, widely distributed and apparently safe drugs. Worldwide production has reached gigantic proportions. Many vitamins are being used for new therapeutic indications, e.g., B-vitamins for mental diseases, E for atherosclerosis, A for skin cancer and acne, pantothenic acid for hair problems, etc. Substantially higher doses have become popular even as dietary supplements and much more so in treatment of mental and neurological disorders and the common cold. Prolonged administration is common practice, e.g., in pregnancy and for growing children who not only get their one-a-day capsule but are vitaminized with their candies, cereals, milk, and other fortified foods. Medical supervision of vitamin intake is virtually non-existant. Thus, a review and a critical appraisal of available safety data of all vitamins would be desirable. Such reviews would almost certainly uncover substantial deficiencies. This opinion is based on my recent attempt to scan the medical literature for animal toxicity data on vitamin C. The most elaborate subacute toxicity study of Na ascorbate in rats was done with female animals only, lasted 10 weeks, included neither blood cell counts nor urinalysis or organ function tests and restricted histological evaluation to liver, heart, and kidney of 7 animals treated with the highest dose (Kieckebusch et al., 1963). I found no long-term toxicity studies with this vitamin. For trials with a second species there were studies on guinea pigs lasting 6 and on mice lasting 7 days (Demole, 1934), and one more with 8 guinea pigs over a period of 42 days (Lamden and Schweiker, 1955). No chronic toxicity studies on subhuman primates are published although this species, like man, and unlike the rat, depends on dietary ascorbic acid. I could not even find any half-way satisfactory teratological experiment with vitamin C, nor any mutagenicity tests done with mammals. There were only two in vitro mutagenicity studies of questionable significance done with plant cells and microorganisms, both showing positive results (Röhrborn, 1965).

From this short summary I conclude that there is indeed a problem to be concerned about. Not that I worry much about toxicity of vitamin C. But what concerns me is the fact that up-dated, modern animal toxicity studies of a drug which is consumed in fantastic quantities are not available to support the safety of a compound whose use has increased so markedly. It is, of course, possible that pharmaceutical companies and government agencies possess additional unpublished toxicity data on ascorbic acid. If this is true, the problem to be concerned about is a different one: That this scientific information is not readily available in the scientific literature.

A Summary of Vitamin Toxicology with Some Newer Findings

The paucity of systematic toxicological studies of vitamins was evident already 10 years ago when we last reviewed the subject (Studer et al., 1962). Recent papers have mostly dealt with certain aspects of the mode of action of the two "toxic" vitamins, A and D. The other vitamins are still considered safe at the doses customarily used. This summary gives the highlights of the 1962 review of Studer et al. without referring to the original literature. It will also include some newer findings.

Vitamin A

Consumption of polar bear liver, explorers have come to know already in the 16th century, can lead to severe skin disease. It is due to chronic hypervitaminosis A, a condition which is still seen in our times as a consequence of overenthusiastic vitamin A therapy. Scaling of the skin may be accompanied by bone pain and swelling of the limbs, due to extensive periostal bone proliferation. Acute vitamin A poisoning, mostly seen in small children, leads to a different syndrome, characterized by increase in intracranial pressure, papilledema, diplopia, pallor, dizziness and vomiting (pseudotumor cerebri, syndrome of Marie and Sée). To the experimental toxicologist A-hypervitaminosis provides the opportunity to enjoy a wide spectrum of bone pathology. In rats, for example, he finds multiple fractures of the limbs with periostal and endostal proliferations and osteolytic processes. Enchondral ossification is accelerated and hyperostoses may develop at the calvaria. Early signs of A-hypervitaminosis in rats include elevated alkaline phosphatase, increase in liver glycogen, elevation of plasma free fatty acids, blood lactic acid and glucose levels and lowering of glucose tolerance (Singh et al., 1968). In other organs one finds less characteristic changes, notably hemorrhages and cell necrosis. Hepatosplenomegaly with functional and morphological signs of liver cell injury is also occasionally seen in man (Rubin et al., 1970). The elevation of alkaline phosphatase, however, is due to increased osteoblastic activity (Ammann et al., 1968). Skin histology is distinguished by marked thickening of the epidermis with acanthosis. In guinea pigs, A-hypervitaminosis caused lymphoreticular proliferation with appearance of atypical mononuclear cells in spleen, liver, lymph nodes and bone marrow (Polliack and Drexler, 1972). The teratological effects of vitamin A with malformations mostly in the cranial region are well documented. Retinoic acid, a form of vitamin A, currently used for topical treatment of acne, was reported to have a greater teratogenic potency than retinyl acetate (Kochhar, 1967). Topical administration to pregnant rats and rabbits, however at maximally tolerated concentrations failed to induce malformations of the offspring. Resorption studies with C^{14} labeled retinoic acid in man showed that considerably less than the recommended daily dose of vitamin A was absorbed through the skin after administration of 1 g of a 0.1% preparation. Because of a marked irritant effect, higher doses could not be tolerated (Hanisch, personal communication). Overuse of this dosage form is therefore impossible. I conclude that topical retinoic acid formulations represent less of a teratogenic hazard to man than high-potency oral vitamin preparations.

The fact that vitamin A causes tissue damage in many organs indi-cates that it may affect an element common to many cell types, most probably the lysosome. Vitamin A was shown to release proteolytic enzymes and acid phosphatase from isolated lysosomes. The same oc-curred in cell cultures, notably those of cartilage, where dissolution of the matrix with release of chondroic acid was observed (Roels, 1969). That this also happens in vivo was documented by the sad picture of a vitamin A-treated rabbit whose ears became limp because their cartilagineous support had melted (Thomas et al., 1960). A-hyper-vitaminosis in mice caused a decrease in acid phosphatase reaction in Kupffer and liver cells (Riecken et al., 1967). If guinea pigs were injected i.p. simultaneously with mineral oil and vitamin A the macro-phages which accumulated in the peritoneal cavity were found to have a reduced content of acid phosphatase (Janoff and McCluskey, 1962). In children a single dose of 200,000 IU of vitamin A often induced an increase in urine aryl sulfatase and acid phosphatase which is thought to be a consequence of enzyme release from lysosomes (Reddy and Mohanram, 1971).

These and other experiments explain why vitamin A has become the beloved standard agent of lysosomists for whom it has proven to be a most welcome bonus. One should not, however, overlook vitamin A's action on other membrane structures. There is evidence that it also affects mitochondria and it probably also damages membrane of erythro-cytes (Roels, 1969). Lysosomal damage is therefore only one of seve-ral points of attack of vitamin A toxicity. In contrast to vitamin A, overdosage with the provitamin, β -carotin, is innocuous. Cows, for example absorb it readily from their feed. It circulates in the blood and gives butter the appetizing yellow tint. In humans, resorption from the gut is limited. One needs to consume enormous amounts of carrots to provoke a yellow discoloration of the adipose tissue and the skin. This carotin icterus is harmless and does not lead to A-hypervitaminosis. Because of its use as a food color, β -carotin was nevertheless tested extensively in multigeneration toxicity stu-dies. They confirmed that Nature's own colors, this one at least, were safe (Zbinden and Studer, 1958; Bagdon et al., 1960).

Vitamin D

Because of heroic attempts to cure rickets with excessively high doses of vitamin D, the toxic effects of this compound in man became all too well known shortly after its discovery. The predominant symptoms are hypercalcemia, and metastatic calcifications. The lesions are predominantly located in the kidneys. Calcium salts are deposited in the epithelium of the proximal convoluted tubules and in the tubular lumen, leading to tubular necrosis, obstruction and renal failure. One also finds calcifications in the gastric mucosa, lungs, skin, and arterial walls. An impressive calcification of the elastic fibers of the aorta is easily produced in rabbits. High single doses caused acceleration of acid mucopolysaccharide synthesis in rat heart and aorta. This represents a change of the mesenchymal tissue which facilitates calcification (Rave et al., 1970). In bones phospholipids were found to be markedly increased, indicating another interesting metabolic effect of vitamin D (Cruess and Clark, 1967). It has recent-ly also been recognized that some children, owing to an inborn meta-bolic error, may be hyperreactive to vitamin D administration.

Evidence is now accumulating that this hyperreactivity may be responsible for a variety of pathological conditions including hypercalcemia of infancy, supravalvular aortic stenosis, mental retardation, tubular acidosis and general arterial calcinosis in infancy (Seelig, 1969; Taussig, 1966).

Vitamin K

This fat soluble vitamin does not produce a specific hypervitaminosis syndrome, and even in high doses it is well tolerated by animals. Less harmless are the water soluble vitamin K surrogates, the menadione derivatives. In animal experiments they were shown to produce hemolysis, methemoglobinemia and Heinz-Ehrlich bodies. Hemolytic anemia was also caused in human newborns who were treated with generous but apparently unnecessarily high doses of these agents. Thus, menadione and its derivatives should be retired to the status of experimental tools and be replaced, at least for the treatment of hypoprothrombinemia, by vitamin K_1 preparations (Zbinden et al., 1957).

Vitamin E

One does not have to be a clairvoyant to predict that this vitamin is at the threshold of a worldwide sales boom. Some years ago it had only a modest success when it was thought to be a fertility vitamin. It is now rumored to prevent ageing and is already consumed regularly by many of my contemporaries. Can we assure them that their new habit, if it is not making them young again, will at least not be harmful? The old literature reviewed in 1962 (Studer et al.) showed no acute toxic effects in mice, rats, and dogs, after oral and i.v. administration. Subacute toxicity in rats was limited to 10 doses of 0.5 to 1 g/kg given during a period of 2 months and 10 times 0.1 g/kg p.o. in dogs. In some experiments acceleration of sexual maturation was observed in young rabbits and rats. Rabbits but not guinea pigs showed hyperplasia of the thyroids with histological signs of activation. These findings indicate that large doses of vitamin E are not entirely inert. I have therefore asked my assistant, Mrs. E Roos, to collect the literature on experimental and clinical toxicology of this vitamin. It is certainly not her fault that the search did not uncover any useful information. There were some clinical reports of patients who had taken up to 60 mg tocopherol acetate for about 2 years without apparent side effects (Ernyei, 1966). There also exists a paper about chicks who received 10,000 IU/kg per day and thrived on it (MuCuaig and Motzok, 1970). But chronic toxicity, teratogenicity, mutagenicity and carcinogenicity studies, as far as she could find out, are not reported. It is hoped that those who may have done such experiments, will publish them before long.

Water Soluble Vitamins

Since these compounds are not extensively stored in the body the danger of chronic overdosage appears small. There are a few exceptions where, at least in animal experiments, repeated administration of high doses can induce tissue damage. An interesting example is vitamin B_6 which, after treatment with high doses, caused hind leg paralysis in rats and dogs. Histopathologically, extensive focal damage of the peripheral nerves was found. Degeneration of the dorsal tracts of the spinal cord, the dorsal roots, and the dorsal spinal ganglia were also described (Antopol and Tarlov, 1942). To induce such lesions in rats one needs large doses, about 500 to 1000 mg/kg per day for several days. But at these levels severe neuromuscular deficits due to axonal damage and widespread degeneration of myelin sheath of peripheral nerves developed rapidly (Alder and Zbinden, unpublished). The histopathological changes are not distinguishable from those induced by isoniazid which is thought to be neurotoxic because of its interference with vitamin B_6 metabolism and whose effect can be inhibited by B_6 treatment. There are one or two unconvincing theories why vitamin B_6 overdosage causes neuropathy. A satisfactory explanation, however, has not been found. In human therapy vitamin B_6 is usually given in daily doses up to 50 mg and is rarely used at several hundred mg per day. At these levels the safety margin appears to be sufficient.

High doses of folic acid caused kidney damage in animals, characterized by marked tubular proliferation and mitochondrial degeneration (Torhorst et al., 1970). At therapeutic levels in man no harmful effects have been noted. p-aminobenzoic acid can cause liver and kidney damage when given at excessive doses. This was also seen in human subjects who were thought to gain therapeutic benefit from daily loads of 20 to 25 g.

Vitamin C is generally well tolerated. At high doses it is said to promote diuresis in animals and man. It occasionally induced skin eruptions and electrolyte imbalance in urine and blood. It acidified urine and can thereby delay excretion of acidic drugs, such as aspirin (personal observation). At reasonable doses it is harmless. Its effect on oxalic acid excretion was discussed on pages 51-52.

A dangerous, sometimes lethal, reaction has occasionally occurred after i.v. injection of vitamin B_1. Patients collapsed suddenly with the clinical signs of an anaphylactic shock. The mechanism of this rare side-effect has not been explained. But it is noteworthy that acute shock and death also occurred after i.v. injection in animals. It appeared to be due to a pharmacological effect since it could be prevented by pyruvic acid and phenobarbital pretreatment. Moreover, tolerance was acquired after repeated administration.

Vitamin B_2 was quite extensively tested in animals and proved to be well tolerated. Only at sublethal doses in dogs was kidney failure due to deposition of concrements observed. No significant toxicity is known of pantothenic acid, vitamin B_{12} and biotin. Nicotinic acid has an acute pharmacologic effect on blood vessels leading to unpleasant side effects such as flushing, pruritis and abdominal cramps. Toxic effects such as fatty change of the liver, gastric erosions and petechial hemorrhage of the colon mucosa were seen at very high doses. In man disturbance of liver function may occur.

The short review has shown that water soluble vitamins are generally well tolerated by mammals including man. This is not the case, however, for insects: Oversupply of vitamin B_6, pantothenic, nicotinic or folic acid kills larvae of the housefly, and biotin disrupts fertility of the Mexican fruit fly and the hidebeetle (Cohen and Levinson, 1968).   This is just an incidental reference for those who postulate that toxicological screening does not have to waste expensive mammals but also could often be done with lower animals.

VIII

GEOGRAPHICAL TOXICOLOGY

GENERAL REMARKS

I am writing this to convince myself that the country I live in, its altitude, its winds, and its soil have some determinant influence on the likelihood that I may suffer from a toxic drug reaction. Had I not experienced the surprising amplification of ethanol neurotoxicity on the Jungfraujoch (3454 m), I would seriously question that geography had anything to do with drug toxicity. But geographical toxicology should not only concern itself with altitude and latitude, geology, and meteorology. It must also investigate the circumstances under which drugs are predominantly used in a certain country, the prescribing habits of its physicians and nutrition of its inhabitants, environmental toxins and specific diseases which are more common in a particular part of the earth. These influences must be distinguished from racial factors, genetically determined peculiarities of metabolism and disposition of the indigenous population. This is often difficult to do, unless large segments of the population have emigrated to other lands, have stayed there reasonably close together and can be investigated properly.

Geographical toxicology is a problem-rich field of research. Many of its difficulties are of a semantic nature. Agranulocytosis, for example, does not signify exactly the same thing in every part of the world, and if you investigate what physicians mean when they talk about leukopenia, exfoliative dermatitis, hypotension, Parkinson-like symptoms, toxic hepatitis, etc. you will find surprising differences. How else could one explain the frequent occurrence that one group of investigators studying a new drug finds virtually no side-effects, whereas another one a few hundred miles away using exactly the same chemical in the same dosage surprises us with a long list of toxic reactions? My own experience has been that such differences, although they may appear real at first, tend to disappear with time. If they don't, they are more likely due to differences in the composition of the drug and its pharmaceutical preparation if they are not just a consequence of different patient selection. There will always remain a small number of examples of toxic drug reactions prevalent in a circumscribed geographical area which defy all simple attempts at explanation. Their investigation leaves one often dissatisfied, but careful analysis of such case histories can sharpen our senses for new and unexpected mechanisms by which drugs may interrelate with environmental factors. This can teach us to try a more sophisticated approach to experimental testing of drugs and perhaps lead us to a more judicious use of these complex substances in our patients.

SUBACUTE MYELO-OPTICO-NEUROPATHY (SMON)

A New Disease?

In the late fifties Japanese neurologists were puzzled by the occurrence of an uncommon type of myelo-neuropathy which was usually
preceded by abdominal pain and diarrhea. Soon thereafter an apparent
increase in sporadic cases and an epidemic occurrence of the syndrome
in isolated areas of the country sparked an all-out effort to grasp
the essential features of the disease, to determine its cause, and to
halt its alarming spread.

Is SMON really a new disease? Japanese physicians seemed to be
convinced of it (Kono, 1971) and Western specialists who visited
Japan did not find much evidence to the contrary. And SMON was not a
rarity either: in some parts of Japan the annual incidence rate exceeded 2 per 100,000 population.

Usually preceded by abdominal pain and persistent diarrhea, the
neurological disease called SMON showed an acute or subacute onset
with bilateral sensory disturbances, paresthesias and dysesthesias,
preferentially in the distal parts of the lower limbs. Other frequent
symptoms were deep sensory disturbances, muscle weakness in the legs,
pyramidal signs, and slight neurological symptoms of the upper limbs.
Rare but typical changes included blurred vision and blindness, a
greenish tongue, disturbances of the vegetative nervous system and
psychological alterations. The disease was more frequent in older
patients, particularly females, and rare in children. It developed
slowly, and in about 15% of the patients it led to severe, permanent
neurological deficits. There were no typical changes of blood and
cerebrospinal fluid. A remarkable characteristic was that SMON occurred often in severely ill hospitalized patients with malignant tumors, chronic nephritis, tuberculosis, diabetes, and other chronic
diseases or after operations. One more interesting feature was the
fact that SMON occurred quite often in small epidemics, in families
and institutions, and among workers of a hospital.

In patients dying with SMON, the cause of death was usually related to intercurrent infection and was only rarely thought to be a
consequence of severe damage to the nervous system. The predominant
morphological changes were bilateral, mostly distal demyelination of
the posterior and lateral long tracts of the spinal cord, most frequently Goll's tract, focal destruction of myelin sheath and axons of
spinal nerve roots and peripheral sensory nerves, severe destruction
of dorsal root ganglions, mostly of the lumbosacral region, minimal
to moderate alterations of ganglion cells in the anterior horn of the
spinal cord and in some areas of the medulla oblongata and pons, demyelination of the optic nerve with disintegration of the cells of
the inner ganglion cell layer of the retina, and mild destructive
processes of the sympathetic and parasympathetic nerves. There were
no signs of acute or chronic inflammation, but some gliosis of brain
and spinal cord and often marked multiplication of Schwann cell nu-
clei in peripheral nerves were noted. No consistent or typical
changes were found in the organs outside the nervous system (Shiraki,
1971).

A Japanese Disease?

In 1965 SMON was recognized as a new clinical entity and as a serious public health problem in Japan (Maeda, 1970). The newly diagnosed cases increased from 1172 in 1966 to 1988 in the year 1969. Although it was obvious that comparable outbreaks of myelo-neuropathy had not occurred anywhere else, a worldwide search was instituted to determine whether or not SMON-like diseases had been observed outside Japan. This effort seemed to have been complicated somewhat by the theory that SMON was a toxic reaction to clioquinol, so much so that a history of prolonged intake of this drug became almost an essential prerequisite for the diagnosis of SMON. After careful investigations a small number of cases of myelo-optico-neuropathy was discovered in widely scattered areas of the globe. Only in part of them was the symptomatology similar to that described for SMON. But even assuming that they all represented the same disease as that making the news in Japan, it is clear that the Japanese outbreak of the neurological disorder called SMON had no parallel anywhere in the world and was essentially a problem of Japan, or, to be exact, of certain provinces of Japan.

A Drug-induced Disease?

The etiology of SMON is not known, although all imaginable causes have been thoroughly discussed and investigated (Maeda, 1970; Kono, 1971). The prevalent opinion today is that the disease is in the majority of cases, in some way related to intake of clioquinol (iodo-chloro-8-hydroxyquinoline), a drug making 93% of Entero-Vioform[R] and also contained in many other popular amebicides and gastrointestinal antiseptics.

In discussing this problem, four possibilities must be considered:

1. SMON is due to a direct neurotoxic action of clioquinol.

2. SMON is related to neurotoxic properties of clioquinol but occurs only in predisposed subjects.

3. SMON is due to an interplay of the neurotoxic action of clioquinol with environmental factors.

4. Clioquinol plays no significant part in the etiology of SMON.

I, for one, admit to a bias for the fourth possibility, although the explanation listed under 3 appeals to me too and served as justification to discuss the problem in the chapter "Geographical Toxicology".

Possibility 1 can be dismissed, I think, since there were a significant number (10 to 15%) of authenticated SMON patients who never took the drug. We should leave it at this and not use a history of clioquinol intake as a necessary differential diagnostic criterion to distinguish SMON from other forms of myelo-neuropathy.

Possibilities 1, 2, and 3 imply that clioquinol has substantial neurotoxic properties. To support this argument, Japanese workers have referred to animal experiments, summarized in the review paper of Kono (1971). It reports that symmetrical weakness and paralysis of the hind legs were induced in mice, guinea pigs, rabbits, and chickens, whereas rats and hamsters seemed to be more resistant. Histologically lesions were found in the peripheral nerves but not in the spinal cord. In dogs, cats, and monkeys, however, clioquinol was claimed to have caused peripheral and spinal lesions comparable to those seen in SMON patients (Tateishi et al., 1971, 1972). Similar experiments done in Switzerland (Hess et al., 1972, 1973) failed to produce morphological nerve injuries in dogs treated with very high doses. Careful electrophysiological investigations of peripheral nerves did not reveal any functional abnormalities. A specific tendency of clioquinol to accumulate in nervous tissues was not found (Hess et al., 1973). The positive and negative findings in higher animals are compared in Table 11. This table should not be regarded

TABLE 11

Toxicological Observations with Clioquinol

Positive Findings	Negative Findings
DOG (mongrel)	DOG (beagle)
7-28 x 60-144 mg/kg p.o.	1 x 800, 1 x 1000 mg/kg p.o.
muscle weakness, increased tendon jerks, hind legs.	no signs of neurotoxicity (3)
degenerative changes and demyelination of fasciculus gracilis and cortico-spinal tracts, degeneration of dorsal root ganglia, degeneration of peripheral nerves and optic tract (1)	7 x 1000 mg/kg p.o. (capsules) marked general toxicity, no neuro-toxicity (3)
	10 x 1000 mg/kg p.o. (suspension)
DOG (beagle)	marked general toxicity, no neuro-toxicity (3)
350 to 450 mg/kg p.o. up to 73 days (?)	
same clinical and pathological changes as in mongrels (2)	122 x 30, 100, 300 mg/kg p.o.
	no effect on peripheral nerve function
MONKEY (one animal)	
subtoxic doses	no histological changes of central and peripheral nervous system (3)
degenerative changes of fasciculus gracilis and dorsal root ganglia (1)	
	CAT
CAT (1 animal)	41 x 100 mg/kg followed by 49 x 300 mg/kg
dose similar as in dogs	eye and optic nerve unchanged (4)
changes of nervous system as in dogs (1)	

(1) Tateishi et al., 1971

(2) Tateishi et al., 1972

(3) Hess et al., 1972

(4) Brückner et al., 1970

as the world's first example that geographical toxicology also applies to animal experiments, but it should demonstrate that surprisingly divergent observations can be made in what seem to be quite straightforward routine tests. A hint which could perhaps help to explain the different findings was given by Tateishi et al. (1972) who found that their inbred beagle dogs were 4 to 5 times more resistant against the toxic effect of clioquinol than their mongrels.

It should not take long, however, to obtain confirmatory evidence for or against the existence of true neurotoxic properties of clioquinol. Until further data are in, it serves my bias better to accept the results of Hess et al. (1972, 1973). Possibility number 2, a specific sensitivity of the Japanese race against clioquinol intoxication, is not probable since the drug has been used for many years without causing SMON, even in Japan. Moreover, it would also not explain the regional differences in incidence in Japan as well as the seasonal peaks usually observed in late summer. Thus, there remains the third possibility, an interplay between clioquinol and environmental factors. These environmental influences could be of a chemical nature, e.g., a pollutant in the air, water, or food, another drug, or an impurity in certain batches of clioquinol. It could also be a virus, a possibility favored by a number of Japanese workers and neither confirmed nor definitely refuted up to now (Maeda, 1970). SMON could also be related to nutritional deficiencies such as hypovitaminosis, pernicious anemia, malabsorption. One must also consider a destruction of essential nutrients by a specific food ingredient (antivitamin), the method of food preparation, a flavor, an antioxydant or some other chemical incorporated for specific purposes into the food. More than one environmental factor could be involved. This means that only when all conditions were met would the disease develop. One of the factors could, of course, be clioquinol, but the fact that many SMON patients never took the drug proves that the other influences must be the dominant ones. The importance of contributing factors to the development of SMON is demonstrated by a remarkable clinical observation of Yoshitake and Igata, summarized in English in the review of Kono (1971). These authors gave clioquinol prophylactically to 78 patients after abdominal surgery and 34 of them came down with SMON within 1 to 3 weeks. 77 patients who did not receive the drug also did not develop neurological disease. This dramatic example of an unusual reaction of a whole patient collective just about proves that an agent must have been present in the hospital which could have been activated by the drug. The nature of this agent remains obscure.

One of the major arguments for a causative role of clioquinol is the observation that after withdrawal of clioquinol in Japan on September 8, 1970, the incidence of SMON fell precipitously (Kono, 1971). Looking at the number of cases newly diagnosed every month, it is evident that it had already dropped in August to a three year low, a tendency which continued right through October. This compared to the previous 3 years where the peak incidence was reached in August or September. Thus the claim that SMON disappeared after withdrawal of clioquinol from the market is not fully supported by the statistics.

These arguments are of course not listed in an attempt to force a supreme judgement for or against clioquinol, but they are presented as an example of the difficulties with which the health authorities and their toxicological advisors are confronted in the face of an obscure but urgent public health problem. Here as in other cases, it was just not possible to let the experiment go on, even though the decision to withdraw clioquinol from the market may have made it impossible to ever learn what really caused the disease SMON.

Postcript

In the introduction to this chapter I wrote that the occupation with geographical toxicology often leaves one dissatisfied. At least in this respect the example of SMON was an appropriate selection. It has taught us, among other things, that there are many unsolved problems left in toxicology.

On July 13, 1917, Paul Klee wrote in his diary: "... es gibt nichts Kritischeres als am Ziel zu sein." Don't worry, friend, we toxicologists still have a long way to go.

ACKNOWLEDGMENT

I thank Mrs. E. Roos and Miss E. Dusablon who helped with the literature research and typed the manuscript.

REFERENCES

Abraham, R., Dougherty, W., Golberg, L., and Coulston, F. (1971). The response of the hypothalamus to high doses of monosodium glutamate in mice and monkeys. Cytochemistry and ultrastructural study of lysosomal changes. Exper. Molec. Pathol. 15, 43-60.

Abraham, S.V. and Teller, J.J. (1969). Influence of various miotics on cataract formation. Brit. J. Ophthal. 53, 833-838.

Adlercreutz, H., Eisalo, A., Heino, A., Luukkainen, T., Penttilä, I., and Saukkonen, H. (1968). Investigations on the effect of an oral contraceptive and its components on liver function, serum proteins, copper, coeruloplasmin and gamma-glutamyl peptidase in post-menopausal women. Scand. J. Gastroent. 3, 273-284.

Allen, J.R. and Chesney, C.F. (1972). Effect of age on development of cor pulmonale in nonhuman primates following pyrrolizidine alkaloid intoxication. Exp. Molec. Pathol. 17, 220-232.

Ammann, P., Herwig, K., and Baumann, T. (1968). Beitrag zur A-Hypervitaminose. Helv. Paed. Acta 23, 137-146.

Anton, A.H. (1968). The effect of disease, drugs, and dilution on the binding of sulfonamides in human plasma. Clin. Pharmac. Ther. 9, 561-567.

Anton, A.H. and Corey, W.T. (1971). Interindividual differences in the protein binding of sulfonamides. The effect of disease and drugs. Acta. Pharmac. Tox. 29, Suppl. 3, 134-151.

Antopol, W. and Tarlov, I.M. (1942). Experimental study of the effects produced by large doses of vitamin B_6. J. Neuropath. exp. Neurol. 1, 330-336.

Asatoor, A.M. (1964). Pyridoxine deficiency in the rat produced by D-penicillamine. Nature 203, 1382-1383.

Astwood, E.B. (1943). The chemical nature of compounds which inhibit the function of the thyroid gland. J. Pharmacol. exp. Ther. 78, 79-89.

Atkins, G.L., Dean, B.M., Griffin, W.J., Scowen, E.F., and Watts, R.W.E. (1965). Quantitative aspects of ascorbic acid metabolism in patients with primary hyperoxaluria. Clin. Sci. 29, 305-314.

Averbukh, E.S. and Lapin, I.P. (1969). Psychiatric and pharmacologic aspects of some peculiarities of effects of antidepressants in the aged. Pharmakopsychiat. Neuro-Psychopharmakol. 2, 88-92.

Bagdon, R.E., Zbinden, G., and Studer, A. (1960). Chronic toxicity studies of β-carotene. Toxicol. appl. Pharmacol. 2, 225-236.

Balazs, T., Murphy, J.B., and Grice, H.C. (1962). The influence of environmental changes on the cardiotoxicity of isoprenaline in rats. J. Pharm. Pharmacol. 14, 740-755.

Baker, E.M., Sauberlich, H.E., Wolfskill, S.J., Wallace, W.T., and Dean, E.E. (1962). Tracer studies of Vitamin C utilization in men: metabolism of D-glucuronolactone-6-C[14], D-glucuronic-6-C[14] acid and L-ascorbic-1-C[14] acid. Proc. Soc. Exp. Biol. Med. 109, 737-741.

Barnes, J.M. and Denz, F.A. (1954). Experimental methods used in determining chronic toxicity. Pharmacol. Rev. 6, 191-242.

Barrett, D.A., II, Dalldorf, F.G., Barnwell, W.H., II, and Hudson, R.P. (1971). Allergic giant cell myocarditis complicating tuberculosis chemotherapy. Arch. Path. 91, 201-205.

Batzenschlager, A., Rousselot, P., et Hennequin, J.P. (1970). Lésions myocardiques et rénales d'hypersensitivité. Path. europ. 5, 105-120.

Bellet, S., Feinberg, L.J., Sandberg, H., and Hirabayashi, M. (1968). The effects of caffeine on free fatty acids and blood coagulation parameters of dogs. J. Pharmacol. exp. Ther. 159, 250-254.

Bianchine, J.R. and Ferguson, F.C., Jr. (1967). Acute toxicity and lethal brain concentration of pentobarbital in young and adult albino rats. Proc. Soc. Exp. Biol. Med. 124, 1077-1079.

Bickel, G. (1960). Allergie et myocarde. Schweiz. med. Wchschr. 90, 912-921.

Binder, M.J., Gunderson, H.J., Cannon, J., and Rosove, L. (1950). Electrocardiographic changes associated with allergic reactions to penicillin. Amer. Heart J. 40, 940-944.

Bliss, C.I. (1935). The calculation of the dosage-mortality curve. Ann. Appl. Biol. 22, 134-167.

Bloom, W.L. (1967). Blood vessel binding of free fatty acid and venous thrombosis. Metabolism 16, 777-786.

Borga, O., Azarnoff, D.L., and Sjöqvist, F. (1968). Species differences in the plasma protein binding of desipramine. J. Pharm. Pharmacol. 20, 571.

Botti, R.E. and Ratnoff, O.D. (1963). The clot-promoting effect of soaps of long-chain saturated fatty acids. J. Clin. Invest. 42, 1569-1577.

Brodie, B.B. (1965). Displacement of one drug by another from carrier or receptor sites. Proc. R. Soc. Med. 58, 946-955.

Brodie, B.B., Cho, A.K., Krishna, G., and Reid, W.D. (1971). Drug metabolism in man: past, present, and future. Ann. N.Y. Acad. Sci. 179, 11-18.

Brownlee, K.A., Hodges, J.L., Jr., and Rosenblatt, M. (1953). The up-and-down method with small samples. J. Amer. Statist. Ass. 48, 262-277.

Brückner, R., Hess, R., Pericin, C., and Tripod, J. (1970). Tierexperimentelle Untersuchungen bei langdauernder Verabreichung von hohen Dosen von Iod-chlor-8-hydroxychinolin mit besonderer Berücksichtigung möglicher toxischer Augenveränderungen. Arzneimittelforsch. 20, 575-577.

Burmeister, W. (1970). Clinical pharmacology in paediatrics. Int. J. Clin. Pharmacol. 4, 32-36.

Burns, J.J., Welch, R.M., and Conney, A.H. (1967). Drug effects on enzymes. In "Animal and Clinical Pharmacologic Techniques in Drug Evaluation". P.E. Siegler and J.H. Moyer, eds. Year Book Medical Publishers Inc. (Chicago) Vol. 2, pp. 67-75.

Busbee, D.L., Shaw, C.R., and Cantrell, E.T. (1972). Aryl hydrocarbon hydroxylase induction in human leukocytes. Science 178, 315-316.

Cammer, W. and Moore, C.L. (1972). The effect of hexachlorophene on the respiration of brain and liver mitochondria. Biochem. Biophys. Res. Commun. 46, 1887-1894.

Carstairs, K.C., Beckenridge, A., Dollery, C.T., and Worlledge, S.M. (1966). Incidence of a positive direct Coombs test in patients on ∝-methyldopa. Lancet 2, 133-135.

Chamberlain, D.A., White, R.J., Howard, M.R., and Smith, T.W. (1970). Plasma digoxin concentrations in patients with atrial fibrillation. Brit. Med. J. 3, 429-432.

Christensen, L.K., Hansen, J.M., Kristensen, M. (1963). Sulphaphena-zole-induced hypoglycaemic attacks in tolbutamide-treated diabetics. Lancet 2, 1298-1301.

Clausen, J. (1966). Binding of sulfonamides to serum proteins: physicochemical and immunochemical studies. J. Pharmacol. Exp. Ther. 153, 167-175.

Cohen, E. and Levinson, H.Z. (1968). Disrupted fertility of the hidebeetle Dermestes maculatus (Deg.) due to dietary overdosage of biotin. Experientia 24, 367-368.

Conney, A.H. (1967). Pharmacological implications of microsomal enzyme induction. Pharmacol. Rev. 19, 317-366.

Conney, A.H. and Burns, J.J. (1972). Metabolic interactions among environmental chemicals and drugs. Science 178, 576-586.

Conney, A.H., Davison, C., Gastel, R., and Burns, J.J. (1960). Adaptive increases in drug-metabolizing enzymes induced by pheno-barbital and other drugs. J. Pharmacol. Exp. Ther. 130, 1-8.

Conney, A.H., Welch, R., Kuntzman, R., Chang, R., Jacobson, M., Munro-Faure, A.D., Peck, A.W., Bye, A., Poland, A., Poppers, P.J., Finster, M., and Wolff, J.A. (1971). Effects of environmental chemicals on the metabolism of drugs, carcinogens and normal body constituents in man. Ann. N.Y. Acad. Sci. 179, 155-172.

Connor, W.E., Hoak, J.C., and Warner, E.D. (1963). Massive thrombo-sis produced by fatty acid infusion. J. Clin. Invest. 42, 860-866.

Conway, J. (1970). Effect of age on the response to propranolol. Int. J. Clin. Pharmacol. 4, 148-150.

Cornfield, J. and Mantel, N. (1950). Some new aspects of the appli-cation of maximum likelihood to the calculation of the dosage response curve. J. Am. Stat. Assoc. 45, 181-210.

Croft, J.D., Jr., Swisher, S.N., Jr., Gilliland, B.C., Bakemeier, R.F., Leddy, J.P., Weed, R.I. (1968). Coombs'-test positivity induced by drugs. Mechanisms of immunologic reactions and red cell destruction. Ann. Intern. Med. 68, 176-187.

Cruess, R.L. and Clark, I. (1967). Effect of hypervitaminosis D upon the phospholipids of metaphyseal and diaphyseal bone. Proc. Soc. Exp. Biol. Med. 126, 8-11.

Curley, A., Hawk, R.E., Kimbrough, R.D., Nathenson, G., and Finberg, L. (1971). Dermal absorption of hexachlorophene in infants. Lancet 2, 296-297.

Dalton, A.C. (1970). Host factors and toxicity of antimicrobial agents. South. Med. J. 63, 858-862.

Davison, A.N. and Dobbing, J. (1966). Myelination as a vulnerable period in brain development. Br. Med. Bull. 22, 40-44.

Dearing, W.H., Barnes, A.R., and Essex, H.E. (1944). Experiments with calculated therapeutic and toxic doses of digitalis. V. Comparative effects of toxic doses of digitalis and of pitressin on the electrocardiogram, heart, and brain. Am. Heart J. 27, 96-107.

DeBeer, E.J. (1945). Calculation of biological assay results by graphic methods. All-or-none type of response. J. Pharmacol. Exp. Ther. 85, 1-13.

Deichmann, W.B. and LeBlanc, T.J. (1943). Determination of the approximate lethal dose with about six animals. J. Ind. Hyg. Toxicol. 25, 415-417.

Deichmann, W.B. and Mergard, E.G. (1948). Comparative evaluation of methods employed to express the degree of toxicity of a compound. J. Ind. Hyg. and Toxicol. 30, 373-378.

Demole, V. (1934). On the physiological action of ascorbic acid and some related compounds. Biochem. J. 28, 770-773.

Depocas, F., Hart, J.S., and Héroux, O. (1957). Energy metabolism of the white rat after acclimation to warm and cold environments. J. Appl. Physiol. 10, 393-397.

Desgrez, P., Thomas, J., and David-Issartel, L. (1968). Contribution à l'étude de l'oxalurie dans la lithiase rénale. Rein Foie 11, 211-220.

Dienemann, G. and Simon, K. (1953). Mitteilung eines Todesfalles nach kombinierter Verabreichung von Irgapyrin und Neoteben (INH). II. (Simon): Tierexperimentelle Untersuchungen zu der vorstehenden Arbeit. Münch. med. Wschr. 95, 221-222.

Dixon, R.L., Henderson, E.S., and Rall, D.P. (1965). Plasma protein binding of methotrexate and its displacement by various drugs. Fed. Proc. 24, 454.

Dixon, W.J. and Mood, A.M. (1948). A method for obtaining and analyzing sensitivity data. J. Am. Stat. Assoc. 43, 109-126.

Djerassi, C. (1969). Prognosis for the development of new chemical birth-control agents. Science 166, 468-473.

Doberenz, A.R., Van Miller, J.P., Green, J.R., and Beaton, J.R. (1971). Vitamin B_6 depletion in women using oral contraceptives as determined by erythrocyte glutamic-pyruvic transaminase activities. Proc. Soc. Exp. Biol. Med. 137, 1100-1103.

Doerr, W., Kraft, A., and Rauschke, J. (1947). Ueber experimentelle Glykolvergiftung. Klin. Wchschr. 24/25, 749-754.

Dyer, R. and Nordin, B.E.C. (1967). Urinary crystals and their relation to stone formation. Nature 215, 751-752.

Ebert, A.G. and Yim, G.K.W. (1961). Barbital sensitivity in the young rat. Toxicol. Appl. Pharmacol. 3, 182-187.

Elliot, J.S. and Ribeiro, M. (1967). Calcium oxalate solubility in urine: the state of relative saturation. Invest. Urol. 5, 239-243.

Ernyei, S. (1966). Allgemeinbehandlung des primären Glaukoms mit Vitamin E (Ein therapeutischer Vorschlag). Klin. Monatsbl. Augenheilkd. 148, 417-422.

European Society for the Study of Drug Toxicity (D.G. Davey) (1965).
The study of the toxicity of a potential drug: basic principles
Proc. Europ. Soc. Study Drug Tox. 6, (Suppl.) 1-13. Internat.
Congress Series No. 97A, Excerpta Medica Foundation.

Fass, R.J., Perkins, R.L., and Saslow, S. (1970). Positive direct
Coombs' tests associated with cephaloridine therapy. JAMA 213,
121-123.

Finney, D.J. (1964). Statistical method in biological assay. 2nd ed.
Charles Griffin and Co. Ltd., London.

Fisher, R.A. (1935). The case of zero survivors (Appendix to Bliss,
1935). Ann. Appl. Biol. 22, 164-165.

Fouts, J.R. and Adamson, R.H. (1959). Drug metabolism in the newborn rabbit. Science 129, 897-898.

Fregly, M.J. (1968). Effect of aminotriazole on thyroid function in
the rat. Toxicol. Appl. Pharmacol. 13, 271-286.

Fuhrman, G.J. and Fuhrman, F.A. (1961). Effects of temperature on
the action of drugs. Ann. Rev. Pharmacol. 1, 65-78.

Fujii, K., Jaffe, H., and Epstein, S.S. (1968). Factors influencing
the hexobarbital sleeping time and zoxazolamine paralysis time in
mice. Toxicol. Appl. Pharmacol. 13, 431-438.

Gardocki, J.F., Schuler, M.E., and Goldstein, L. (1966). Reconsidera-
tion of the central nervous system pharmacology of amphetamine.
I. Toxicity in grouped and isolated mice. Toxicol. Appl. Pharmacol.
8, 550-557.

Gehring, P.J. and Buerge, J.F. (1969). The cataractogenic activity
of 2,4-dinitrophenol in ducks and rabbits. Toxicol. Appl. Pharmacol. 14, 475-486.

Geiling, E.M.K. and Cannon, R.R. (1938). Pathologic effects of
elixir of sulfanilamide (diethylene glycol) poisoning. A clinical
and experimental correlation: final report. JAMA 111, 919-926.

Gelboin, H.V., Wortham, J.S., and Wilson, R.G. (1967). 3-methylcho-
lanthrene and phenobarbital stimulation of rat liver RNA polymerase.
Nature, 214, 281-283.

Gershoff, S.N. and Faragalla, F.F. (1959). Endogenous oxalate
synthesis and glycine, serine, deoxypyridoxine interrelationships
in vitamin B_6-deficient rats. J. Biol. Chem. 234, 2391-2393.

Gillette, J.R. (1971). Factors affecting drug metabolism. Ann. N.Y.
Acad. Sci. 179, 43-66.

Gleason, M.N., Gosselin, R.E., Hodge, H.C., and Smith, R.P. (1969).
Clinical toxicology of commercial products. Acute Poisoning.
3rd ed. Williams and Williams, Baltimore, Md.

Goldenthal, E.I. (1966). Guidelines for reproduction studies for
safety evaluation of drugs for human use. A Communication of the
FDA, January 1966.

Goldenthal, E.I. (1968). Current views on safety evaluation of
drugs. FDA Papers 2, May, 1-8.

Goldenthal, E.I. (1969). Contraceptives, estrogens, and progestogens: A new FDA policy on animal studies. FDA Papers, 3, Novem-
ber, 15.

Goldenthal, E.I. (1971). A compilation of LD_{50} values in newborn and adult animals. Toxicol. Appl. Pharmacol. 18, 185-207.

Gralnick, H.R., Wright, L.D. Jr., and McGinniss, M.H. (1967). Coombs' positive reactions associated with sodium cephalothin therapy. JAMA 199, 725-726.

Gram, T.E., Schroeder, D.H., Davis, D.C., Reagan, R.L. and Guarino, A.M. (1971). Enzymic and biochemical composition of smooth and rough microsomal membranes from monkey, guinea pig and mouse liver. Biochem. Pharmacol. 20, 1371-1381.

Gray, J.E., Purmalis, A., and Mulvihill, W.J. (1966). Further toxicologic studies with lincomycin. Toxicol. Appl. Pharmacol. 9, 445-454.

Grogan, D.E., Lane, M., Smith, F.E., Bresnick, E., and Stone, K. (1972). Interaction of flavins and chloramphenicol with microsomal enzyme systems. Biochem. Pharmacol. 21, 3131-3144.

Gump, W.S. (1969). Toxicological properties of hexachlorophene. J. Soc. Cosmetic Chemists 22, 173-184.

Hall, G.E., Ettinger, G.H., and Banting, F.G. (1936). An experimental production of coronary thrombosis and myocardial failure. Can. Med. Assoc. J. 34, 9-15.

Hansen, A.R. and Fouts, J.R. (1968). Influence of 3,4-benzpyrene or gamma-chlordane on the rate of metabolism and acute toxicity of aminopyrine, hexobarbital, and zoxazolamine in the mouse. Toxicol. Appl. Pharmacol. 13, 212-219.

Hansen, J.M., Kristensen, M., Skovsted, L., and Christensen, L.K. (1966). Dicoumarol-induced diphenylhydantoin intoxication. Lancet 2, 265-266.

Harrison, Y.E. and West, W.L. (1971). Stimulatory effect of charcoal-broiled ground beef on the hydroxylation of 3,4-benzpyrene by enzymes in rat liver and placenta. Biochem. Pharmacol. 20, 2105-2108.

Haskell, C.M., Canellos, G.P., Leventhal, B.G. Carbone, P.P., Block, J.B., Serpick, A.A., and Selawry, O.S. (1969). L-asparaginase. Therapeutic and toxic effects in patients with neoplastic disease. N. Engl. J. Med. 281, 1028-1034.

Hebold, G. (1972). Guidelines for the testing of drugs in various countries. Proceedings of the VIII World Congress of Anatomic and Clinical Pathology. Munich, 12-16 September 1972, Excerpta Medica, Amsterdam, the Netherlands, in press.

Hedinger, Chr. and Egloff, B. (1967). Normale und pathologische Anatomie der Schilddrüse. In "Die Krankheiten der Schilddrüse". K. Oberdisse and E. Klein, eds. Georg Thieme Verlag, Stuttgart. pp. 6-49.

Hess, R., Keberle, H., Koella, W.P., Schmid, K., and Gelzer, J. (1972). Clioquinol: absence of neurotoxicity in laboratory animals. Lancet 2, 424-425.

Hess, R., Koella, W.P., Krinke, G., Petermann, H., Thomann, P., and Zak, F. (1973). Absence of neurotoxicity following prolonged administration of Iodochloro-8-hydroxyquinoline (Entero-Vioform[R]) to beagle dogs. Arzneimittelforsch. in press

Hoak, J.C., Poole, J.C.F., and Robinson, D.S. (1963). Thrombosis associated with mobilization of fatty acids. Am. J. Path. 43, 987-998.

Hoak, J.C., Warner, E.D., and Connor, W.E. (1966). Platelet aggregation and fatty acids. Thromb. Diath. Haemorrh. 15, 635-636.

Hodgkinson, A. and Zarembski, P.M. (1968). Oxalic acid metabolism in man: a review. Calcif. Tissue Res. 2, 115-132.

Holtz, P. and Palm, D. (1964). Pharmacological aspects of vitamin B_6. Pharmacol. Rev. 16, 113-178.

Hoogland, D.R., Miya, T.S., and Bousquet, W.F. (1966). Metabolism and tolerance studies with chlordiazepoxide-2-^{14}C in the rat. Toxicol. Appl. Pharmacol. 9, 116-123.

Hudson, R.H., Tucker, R.K., and Haegele, M.A. (1972). Effect of age on sensitivity: acute oral toxicity of 14 pesticides to mallard ducks of several ages. Toxicol. Appl. Pharmacol. 22, 556-561.

Jaffe, I.A., Altman, K., and Merryman, P. (1964). The antipyridoxine effect of penicillamine in man. J. Clin. Invest. 43, 1869-1873.

Janoff, A. and McCluskey, R.T. (1962). Effect of excess vitamin A on acid phosphatase content of guinea pig peritoneal leucocytes. Proc. Soc. Exp. Biol. Med. 110, 586-589.

Jondorf, W.R., Maickel, R.P., and Brodie, B.B. (1959). Inability of newborn mice and guinea pigs to metabolize drugs. Biochem. Pharmacol. 1, 352-354.

Kalser, S.C., Evans, D., Forbes, E., Kelly, M., Kelvington, E., Kunig, R., and Randolph, M. (1967). Decreased atropine toxicity in rats chronically exposed to cold. Toxicol. Appl. Pharmacol. 11, 511-522.

Kang, L. and DaVanzo, J.P. (1966). Is the tryptophan load test a valid index for a chemically-induced vitamin B_6 deficiency? Proc. Soc. Exp. Biol. Med. 123, 340-343.

Kato, R., Chiesara, E., and Frontino, G. (1961). Induced increase of meprobamate metabolism in rats pretreated with phenobarbital or phenaglycodol in relation to age. Experientia 17, 520-521.

Kato, R., Takanaka, A., and Shoji, H. (1969). Inhibition of drug-metabolizing enzymes of liver microsomes by hydrazine derivatives in relation to their lipid solubility. Jap. J. Pharmacol. 19, 315-322.

Kavetsky, R.E., Turkevich, N.M., Akimova, R.N., Khayetsky, I.K., and Matveichuck, Y.D. (1969). Induced carcinogenesis under various influences on the hypothalamus. Ann. N.Y. Acad. Sci. 164, 517-519.

Kieckebusch, W., Griem, W., and Lang, K. (1963). Untersuchungen über die chronische Toxizität der Ascorbinsäure bei der Ratte. Z. Ernaehrungswiss. 4, 5-14.

Kimbrough, R.K. (1971). Review of the toxicity of hexachlorophene. Arch. Environ. Health 23, 119-122.

Kimbrough, R.D. and Gaines, T.B. (1971). Hexachlorophene effects on the rat brain. Study of high doses by light and electron microscopy. Arch. Environ. Health 23, 114-118.

Klinge, O. (1966). Charcot-Leydensche Kristalle und Riesenzellen bei akuter, eosinophiler Myocarditis. Beitr. Path. Anat. 133, 297-312.

Kochhar, D.M. (1967). Teratogenic activity of retinoic acid. Acta Pathol. Microbiol. Scand. 70, 398-404.

Kolmodin, B., Azarnoff, D.L., and Sjöqvist, F. (1969). Effect of environmental factors on drug metabolism: Decreased plasma half-life of antipyrine in workers exposed to chlorinated hydrocarbon insecticides. Clin. Pharmacol. Ther. 10, 638-642.

Kono, R. (1971). Subacute myelo-optico-neuropathy, a new neurological disease prevailing in Japan. Jap. J. Med. Sci. Biol. 24, 195-216.

Kuchinskas, E.J. and duVigneaud, V. (1957). An increased vitamin B_6 requirement in the rat on a diet containing L-penicillamine. Arch. Biochem. Biophys. 66, 1-9.

Kunin, C.M. (1967). Clinical significance of protein binding of the penicillins. Ann. N.Y. Acad. Sci. 145, 282-289.

Kupferberg, H.J. and Way, E.L. (1963). Pharmacologic basis for the increased sensitivity of the newborn rat to morphine. J. Pharmacol. Exp. Ther. 141, 105-112.

Lamden, M.P. and Chrystowski, G.A. (1954). Urinary oxalate excretion by man following ascorbic acid ingestion. Proc. Soc. Exp. Biol. Med. 85, 190-192.

Lamden, M.P. and Schweiker, C.E. (1955). Effects of prolonged massive administration of ascorbic acid to guinea pig. Fed. Proc. 14, 439-440.

Lee, C.C. (1966). Comparative pharmacologic responses to antihistamines in newborn and young rats. Toxicol. Appl. Pharmacol. 8, 210-217.

Lehman, A.J. (1959). Newer trends in the laboratory evaluation of the safety of drugs. Bull. Parenter. Drug Assoc. 13, 2-6.

Lehman, A.J. (1963). The intent of the preclinical assessment of new drugs. Joint Symposium on Safety Evaluation of New Drugs, sponsored by A.M.A. Sect. of Exper. Med. Therap. and the Society of Toxicology, Atlantic City, N.J. June 17, 1963.

Lehman, A.J., Patterson, W.I., Davidow, B., Hagan, E.C., Woodard, G., Laug, E.P., Frawley, J.P., Fitzhugh, O.G., Bourke, A.R., Draize, J.H., Nelson, A.A., and Vos, B.J. (1955). Procedures for the appraisal of the toxicity of chemicals in foods, drugs and cosmetics. Food Drug Cosmetic Law J. 10, 679-748.

Levin, W., Conney, A.H., Alvares, A.P. Merkatz, I., and Kappas, A. (1972). Induction of benzol [∝] pyrene hydroxylase in human skin. Science 176, 419-420.

Levin, W., Welch, R.M., and Conney, A.H. (1968). Effect of phenobarbital and other drugs on the metabolism and uterotropic action of estradiol-17β and estrone. J. Pharmacol. Exp. Ther. 159, 362-371.

Lischner, H., Seligman, S.J., Krammer, A., and Parmelee, A.H., Jr. (1961). An outbreak of neonatal deaths among term infants associated with administration of chloramphenicol. J. Pediatr. 59, 21-34.

Litchfield, J.T., Jr. and Wilcoxon, F. (1949). A simplified method of evaluating dose-effect experiments. J. Pharmacol. Exp. Ther. 96, 99-113.

LoBuglio, A.F. and Jandl, J.H. (1967). The nature of the alpha-methyldopa red-cell antibody. N. Engl. J. Med. 276, 658-665.

Lockhart, J.D. (1972). How toxic is hexachlorophene? Pediatrics 50, 229-235.

Luhby, A.L., Brin, M., Gordon, M., Davis, P., Murphy, M., and Spiegel, H. (1971). Vitamin B_6 metabolism in users of oral contraceptive agents. 1. Abnormal urinary xanthurenic acid excretion and its correction by pyridoxine. Am. J. Clin. Nutr. 24, 684-693.

Maeda, K. (1970). Encephalomyelopathy following abdominal symptoms: epidermiological and follow-up studies, histological changes of Auerbach's plexus, and urinary porphyrin. Mie Med. J. 19, 209-233.

McChesney, E.W., Conway, W.D., Braemer, A.C., and Koss, R.F. (1969). Metabolism of nalidixic acid in the calf: the effect of age. Toxicol. Appl. Pharmacol. 14, 138-150.

Menzer, R.E. and Best, N.H. (1968). Effect of phenobarbital on the toxicity of several organophosphorus insecticides. Toxicol. Appl. Pharmacol. 13, 37-42.

Miller, L.C. and Tainter, M.L. (1944). Estimation of the ED_{50} and its error by means of logarithmic-probit graph paper. Proc. Soc. Exp. Biol. Med. 57, 261-264.

Molthan, L., Reidenberg, M.M., and Eichman, M.T. (1967). Positive direct Coombs tests due to cephalothin. N. Engl. J. Med. 277, 123-125.

MuCuaig, L.W. and Motzok, I. (1970). Excessive dietary vitamin E: Its alleviation of hypervitaminosis A and lack of toxicity. Poult. Sci. 49, 1050-1052.

National Cancer Institute (1969). General Protocol for Preclinical Toxicology, Laboratory of Toxicology. Courtesy of Dr. D.P. Rall.

Nebert, D.W., Goujon, F.M., and Gielen, J.E. (1972). Aryl hydrocarbon hydroxylase induction by polycyclic hydrocarbons: Simple autosomal dominant trait in the mouse. Nature (New Biology) 236, 107-110.

Newbould, B.B. and Kilpatrick, R. (1960). Long-acting sulphonamides and protein-binding. Lancet I, 887-891.

Page, J.G. and Vesell, E.S. (1969). Hepatic drug metabolism in ten strains of Norway rat before and after pretreatment with phenobarbital. Proc. Soc. Exp. Biol. Med. 131, 256-261.

Paulini, K., Beneke, G., and Kulka, R. (1971). Zytophotometrische und autoradiographische Untersuchungen zur Lebervergrösserung nach Phenobarbital in Abhängigkeit vom Lebensalter. Beitr. Pathol. 144, 319-326.

Peck, H.M. (1968). An appraisal of drug safety evaluation in animals and the extrapolation of results to man. In "Importance of Fundamental Principles in Drug Evaluation." D. H. Tedeschi and R.E. Tedeschi, eds. Raven Press, New York. pp. 449-471.

Pines, W.L. (1972). Hexachlorophene: Why FDA concluded that hexachlorophene was too potent and too dangerous to be used as it once was. FDA Consumer 6, 24-27.

Plueckhahn, V.D. and Banks, J. (1972). Hexachlorophene toxicity, the new-born child and the staphylococcus. Med. J. Aust. 1, 897-903.

Polliack, A. and Drexler, R. (1972). A light and electron microscopic study of the lymphomyeloid complex in hypervitaminosis A. Blood 40, 528-541.

Randall, L.O., Bagdon, R.E., and Engelberg, R. (1959). Toxicologic and metabolic studies on 2,4-dimethoxy-6-sulfanilamide-1,3-diazine (Madribon). Toxicol. Appl. Pharmacol. 1, 28-37.

Raskin, N.H. and Fishman, R.A. (1965). Pyridoxine-deficiency neuropathy due to hydralazine. N. Engl. J. Med. 273, 1182-1185.

Rave, O., Wagner, H., Hüther, W., Junge-Hülsing, G., and Hauss, W.H. (1970). Risiko der Vitamin-D-Stossprophylaxe. Untersuchungen über den Einfluss des Vitamin D auf den Stoffwechsel der sulfatierten Mukopolysaccharide des Bindegewebes. Münch. Med. Wchschr. 112, 16-21.

Reddy, V. and Mohanram, M. (1971). Urinary excretion of lysosomal enzymes in hypovitaminosis and hypervitaminosis A in children. Int. J. Vitam. Nutr. Res. 41, 321-326.

Remmer, H. and Merker, H.J. (1963). Drug-induced changes in the liver endoplasmic reticulum: Association with drug-metabolizing enzymes. Science 142, 1657-1658.

Reuber, M.D. (1967). Hepatic lesions in young rats given calcium disodium edetate. Toxicol. Appl. Pharmacol. 11, 321-326.

Richardson, K.E. (1967). Effects of vitamin B_6, glycolic acid, testosterone, and castration on the synthesis, deposition, and excretion of oxalic acid in rats. Toxicol. Appl. Pharmacol. 10, 40-53.

Riecken, E.O., Gössner, W., and Pearse, A.G.E. (1967). Akute Vitamin A-intoxikation der Maus. Frühveränderungen an der histochemisch nachweisbaren unspezifischen sauren Phosphatase in Dünndarm und Leber. Histochemie 8, 22-33.

Roels, O.A. (1969). The influence of vitamins A and E on lysosomes. In "Lysosomes in Biology and Pathology". Vol. 1. J.T. Dingle and H.B. Fell, eds. North-Holland Publishing Co., Amsterdam-London. pp. 254-275.

Röhrborn, G. (1965). Ueber mögliche mutagene Nebenwirkungen von Arzneimitteln beim Menschen. Humangenetik 1, 205-231.

Rona, G., Chappel, C.I., Balazs, T., and Gaudry, R. (1959). The effect of breed, age, and sex on myocardial necrosis produced by isoproterenol in the rat. J. Gerontol. 14, 169-173.

Rose, D.P. and Braidman, I.P. (1971). Excretion of tryptophan metabolites as affected by pregnancy, contraceptive steroids, and steroid hormones. Am. J. Clin. Nutr. 24, 673-683.

Rubin, E. Florman, A.L., Degnan, T., and Diaz, J. (1970). Hepatic injury in chronic hypervitaminosis A. Am. J. Dis. Child. 119, 132-138.

Schröpl, F. and Stollmann, K. (1967). Akute, interstitielle eosinophile Myokarditis als ernste Komplikation bei Arzneimittelexanthemen. Münch. Med. Wchschr. 109, 1580-1585.

Schwartz, A. (1968). Ueber die allergische Herzwandentzündung. Beitr. Pathol. Anat. 136, 316-340.

Schwetz, B.A. and Becker, B.A. (1971). Comparison of the lethality of inhaled diethyl ether in neonatal and adult rats. Toxicol. Appl. Pharmacol. 18, 703-706.

Scott, G.L., Myles, A.B., and Bacon, P.A. (1968). Autoimmune haemolytic anemia and mefenamic acid therapy. Br. Med. J. 3, 534-535.

Seelig, M.S. (1969). Vitamin D and cardiovascular, renal, and brain damage in infancy and childhood. Ann. N.Y. Acad. Sci. 147, 539-582.

Sellers, E.M. and Koch-Weser, J. (1971). Kinetics and clinical importance of displacement of warfarin from albumin by acidic drugs. Ann. N.Y. Acad. Sci. 179, 213-225.

Severeid, L., Connor, W.E., and Long, J.P. (1969). The depressant effect of fatty acids on the isolated rabbit heart. Proc. Soc. Exp. Biol. Med. 131, 1239-1243.

Shiraki, H. (1971). Neuropathology of subacute myelo-optico-neuropathy, "SMON". Jap. J. Med. Sci. Biol. 24, 217-243.

Shoeman, D.W. and Azarnoff, D.L. (1972). The alteration of plasma proteins in uremia as reflected in their ability to bind digitoxin and diphenylhydantoin. Pharmacology 7, 169-177.

Singh, M., Singh, V.N., and Venkitasubramanian, T.A. (1968). Early effects of feeding excess vitamin A, hepatic glycogen, blood lactic acid, plasma NEFA and glucose tolerance in rats. Life Sci. 7, 239-247.

Smith, F.A., Downs, W.L., Hodge, H.C., and Maynard, E.A. (1960). Screening of fluorine-containing compounds for acute toxicity. Toxicol. Appl. Pharmacol. 2, 54-58.

Smyth, H.F., Carpenter, C.P., Weil, C.S., Pozzani, U.C., and Striegel, J.A. (1962). Range-finding toxicity data: List VI. Am. Ind. Hyg. Assoc. J. 23, 95-107.

Soffer, A. (1961). The changing clinical picture of digitalis intoxication. Arch. Intern. Med. 107, 681-688.

Stenger, R.J., Miller, R.A., and Williamson, J.N. (1970). Effects of phenobarbital pretreatment on the hepato-toxicity of carbon tetrachloride. Exp. Mol. Pathol. 13, 242-252.

Studer, A., Zbinden, G., and Uehlinger, E. (1962). Die Pathologie der Avitaminosen und Hypervitaminosen. In Handbuch der Allgemeinen Pathologie. F. Büchner, E. Letterer and F. Roulet, eds. Springer Verlag, Berlin, Göttingen, Heidelberg. Vol. II, part 1, pp. 734-1063.

Takenouchi, K., Aso, K., Kawase, K., Ichikawa, H., and Shiomi, T. (1966). On the metabolites of ascorbic acid, especially oxalic acid, eliminated in urine, following the administration of large amounts of ascorbic acid. J. Vitaminol. 12, 49-58.

Taptiklis, N. (1968). Dormancy by dissociated thyroid cells in the lungs of mice. Eur. J. Cancer 4, 59-66.

Taptiklis, N. (1969). Penetration of the vascular endothelial barrier by non-neoplastic thyroid cells in circulation. Eur. J. Cancer 5, 445-457.

Tateishi, J., Kuroda, S., Saito, A., and Otsuki, S. (1971). Myelo-optic neuropathy induced by clioquinol in animals. Lancet 2, 1263-1264.

Tateishi, J., Kuroda, S., Saito, A., and Otsuki, S. (1972). Strain-differences in dogs for neurotoxicity of clioquinol. Lancet 1, 1289-1290.

Taussig, H.B. (1966). Possible injury to the cardiovascular system from vitamin D. Ann. Intern. Med. 65, 1195-1200.

Thomas, L., McCluskey, R.T., Potter, J.L., and Weissmann, G. (1960). Comparison of the effects of papain and vitamin A on cartilage. I. The effects in rabbits. J. Exp. Med. 111, 705-718.

Thompson, W.R. (1947). Use of moving averages and interpolation to estimate median-effective dose. I. Fundamental formulas, estimation of error, and relation to other methods. Bacteriol. Rev. 11, 115-145.

Thorp, J.M. (1964). The influence of plasma proteins on the action of drugs. In Binns, T.B. and Dodds, C., eds. Absorption and Distribution of Drugs. The Williams and Wilkins Company, Baltimore. pp. 64-76.

Tonelli, G. (1966). Acute toxicity of corticosteroids in the rat. Toxicol. Appl. Pharmacol. 8, 250-258.

Torhorst, J., Schmidt, V., and Dubach, U.C. (1970). Veränderungen des Rattennephron nach Folsäure. Verh. Dtsch. Ges. Pathol. 54, 570-574.

Tu, J.B., Blackwell, R.Q., and Lee, P.F. (1963). DL-penicillamine as a cause of optic axial neuritis. JAMA 185, 83-86.

Tuchmann-Duplessis, H. (1972). Teratogenic drug screening. Present procedures and requirements. Teratology 5, 271-285.

Vesell, E.S. and Page, J.G. (1968). Genetic control of drug levels in man: antipyrine. Science 161, 72-73.

Vest, M.F. and Rossier, R. (1963). Detoxification in the newborn: the ability of the newborn infant to form conjugates with glucuronic acid, glycine, acetate and glutathione. Ann. N.Y. Acad. Sci. 111, 183-197.

Vilde, F. and Nezelof, C. (1966). Aspects histo-pathologiques des goitres avec troubles de l'hormonosynthèse. Apropos de 7 observations anatomo-cliniques. Ann. Anat. Pathol. 11, 397-414.

von Sengbusch, R. and Sücker, I. (1966). Bestimmung der Oxalsäure im Urin und die Beeinflussung seines Oxalatgehaltes durch exogene und endogene Faktoren. Z. Klin. Chem. 4, 3-8.

von Sengbusch, R. and Timmermann, A. (1957). Die Bildung von Calciumoxalat-Mikrosteinen im menschlichen Harn und ihre Veränderung durch diätetische und medikamentöse Massnahmen. Urol. Int. 5, 218-231.

Webster, H.D., Johnston, R.L., and Duncan, G.W. (1967). Toxicologic and interrelated studies with an oxazolidinethione contraceptive. Toxicol. Appl. Pharmacol. 10, 322-333.

Weihe, W.H. (1973). The effect of temperature on the action of drugs. Annu. Rev. Pharmacol. 13 (in press).

Weil, C.S. (1952). Tables for convenient calculation of median-effective dose (LD_{50} or ED_{50}) and instructions in their use. Biometrics 8, 249-263.

Weil, C.S. and Wright, G.J. (1967). Intra- and interlaboratory comparative evaluation of single oral test. Toxicol. Appl. Pharmacol. 11, 378-388.

Welch, R.M., Harrison, Y.E., and Burns, J.J. (1967). Implications of enzyme induction in drug toxicity studies. Toxicol. Appl. Pharmacol 10, 340-351.

Wheeler, A.G., Dansby, D., Hawkins, H.C., Payne, H.G., and Weikel, J.H., Jr. (1962). A toxicologic and hematologic evaluation of cyclophosphamide (Cytoxan[R]) in experimental animals. Toxicol. Appl. Pharmacol. 4, 324-343.

WHO (1966). Principles for pre-clinical testing of drug safety. Wld. Hlth. Org. Techn. Rep. Ser. 341.

WHO (1967). Principles for the testing of drugs for Teratogenicity. Wld. Hlth. Org. Techn. Rep. Ser. 364.

WHO (1968). Principles for the clinical evaluation of drugs. Wld. Hlth. Org. Techn. Rep. Ser. 403.

WHO (1969). Principles for the testing and evaluation of drugs for carcinogenicity. Wld. Hlth. Org. Techn. Rep. Ser. 426.

WHO (1971). Evaluation and testing of drugs for mutagenicity: Principles and problems. Wld. Hlth. Org. Techn. Rep. Ser. 482.

Wiberg, G.S., Trenholm, H.L., and Coldwell, B.B. (1970). Increased ethanol toxicity in old rats: Changes in LD_{50}, in vivo and in vitro metabolism, and liver alcohol dehydrogenase activity. Toxicol. Appl. Pharmacol. 16, 718-727.

Worlledge, S.M., Carstairs, K.C., and Dacie, J.V. (1966). Autoimmune haemolytic anaemia associated with α-methyldopa therapy. Lancet 2, 135-139.

Wyngaarden, J.B. and Elder, T.D. (1966). Primary hyperoxaluria and oxalosis. In The Metabolic Basis of Inherited Disease. J.B. Stanbury, J.B. Wyngaarden, and D.J. Fredrickson, eds. 2nd edition. McGraw-Hill Book Company, New York. pp. 189-212.

Yeary, R.A., Benish, R.A., and Finkelstein, M. (1966). Acute toxicity of drugs in newborn animals. J. Pediatr. 69, 663-667.

Zarembski, P.M. and Hodgkinson, A. (1969). Some factors influencing the urinary excretion of oxalic acid in man. Clin. Chim. Acta 25, 1-10.

Zbinden, G. (1963). Experimental and clinical aspects of drug toxicity. Adv. Pharmacol. 2, 1-112.

Zbinden, G. (1964). The problem of the toxicologic examination of drugs in animals and their safety in man. Clin. Pharmacol. Ther. 5, 537-545.

Zbinden, G. (1966a) Modification of the irritant effects of intra-peritoneally administered phenylbutazone in rats after prolonged treatment with the same drug or phenobarbital. Toxicol. Appl. Pharmacol. 9, 319-323.

Zbinden, G. (1966b). The significance of pharmacologic screening tests in the preclinical safety evaluation of new drugs. J. New Drugs 6, 1-7.

Zbinden, G. (1967). Lauric acid-induced thrombocytopenia and thrombosis in rabbits. Thromb. Diath. Haemorrh. 18, 57-65.

Zbinden, G. (1969). Drug Safety: experimental programs. Science 164, 643-647.

Zbinden, G. and Alder, S. (1973). Peripheral neuropathy in hexachlorophene (HCP)-treated rats. Experientia (in press).

Zbinden, G., Mehrishi, J.N., and Tomlin, S. (1970). Assessment of damage to human platelets after aggregation and other injuries by microscopic observation and estimation of serotonin uptake. Thromb. Diath. Haemorrh. 23, 261-275.

Zbinden, G., Schärer, K., and Studer, A. (1957). Experimentelle Untersuchungen über Erythrocytenschädigung durch Menadionderivate im Vergleich zu Vitamin K_1. Schweiz. Med. Wochenschr. 87, 1238-1241.

Zbinden, G. and Studer, A. (1955). Vergleichende Untersuchungen über die Wirkung von Pyridoxin, Pyridoxal-5'-phosphat und Pyridoxalisonicotinyl-hydrazon auf die experimentelle Isoniazid-"Neuritis" der Ratte. Int. Z. Vitforsch. 26, 130-137.

Zbinden, G. and Studer, A. (1956). Einfluss quantitativer Mangelernährung auf Wachstum, Blut und Blutbildung von Ratten verschiedenen Lebensalters. Verh. Naturf. Ges. Basel 67, 341-366.

Zbinden, G. and Studer, A. (1958). Tierexperimentelle Untersuchungen über die chronische Verträglichkeit von β-Carotin, Lycopin, 7,7'-Dihydro-β-carotin und Bixin. Z. Lebensm. Untersuch. Forsch. 108, 113-134.

Zeh, E. and Klaus, D. (1962). Die medikamentös-allergische Myokarditis. Med. Welt 31, 1355-1358.

Ziem, M., Coper, H., Broermann, I., and Strauss, S. (1970). Vergleichende Untersuchungen über einige Wirkungen des Amphetamins bei Ratten verschiedenen Alters. Naunyn-Schmiedebergs. Arch. Pharmak. 267, 208-223.

INDEX

Absorption, 20, 25, 40, 44
Acclimatization, 44
Acetanilide, 40
Acetylcholine, 43
Acrodynia, 37
ACTH, 35
Acute toxicity, 23-27, 39-41
Age, 31, 38-43
Alcohol dehydrogenase, 43
Allergy, 52
Ambient temperature, 43-45
Amidephrine mesylate, 39
p-Aminobenzoic acid, 47, 64
Aminopyrine, 29, 36, 40
Aminosalicylic acid, 53
Aminotriazole, 47
Amphetamine, 25, 26, 40, 42
Anphylactic shock, 53
Antipyrine, 31
Approximate lethal dose method,
  26
Arylhydrocarbon hydroxylase, 32
Ascorbic acid, 29, 51, 52, 60,
  64
L-Asparaginase, 34
Aspirin, 53, 64
Atropin, 44

Barbiturates, 29-31, 41
3,4-Benzpyrene, 29
Benzpyrene hydroxylase, 32
Biotin, 64
Bishydroxycoumarin, 31
Bladder stones, 52
Blood-brain barrier, 41
Blood-aqueous humor barrier, 41
Bone marrow depression, 34

Caffeine, 35, 44
Calcium disodium edetate, 42
Carbamazepine, 53
Carbon tetrachloride, 30
Carbonyl trapping agents, 36
Carcinogenicity, 12-15, 30
β-Carotin, 62
Cephaloridine, 55
Cephalothin, 54, 55
Charcot-Leyden crystals, 53
Chemical information, 20
Chloral hydrate, 34
Chloramphenicol, 30, 39, 40
Chlordane, 29
Chlordiazepoxide, 29

Chlorpheniramine maleate, 40
Chlorpromazine, 40
Chlorpropamide, 47
Chronic toxicity studies, 5-12,
  17-19
Clioquinol, 68-71
CNS depressants, 41
CNS stimulants, 41
Colimycin, 53
Convulsions, 36
Coombs test, 54, 55
Cyanides, 48
Cyclophosphamide, 25
Cycloserine, 36, 37

DDT, 29
Desipramine, 33
Dexamethasone, 24
Diazoxide, 34
Dicoumarol, 30
Diethyl glycol, 50
Diethylether, 41
Digitalis, 43
Dimethoate, 30
Diphenhydramine, 40
Diphenylhydantoin, 30, 31
Discretionary toxicity study,
  10, 11
Drug excretion, 41
Drug interactions, 21, 29-35
Drug metabolizing enzymes, 28-33,
  40

ECG changes, 52, 53
Elixir sulfanilamide, 50
Encephalopathy, 57, 58
Endocrine investigations, 22
Endoplasmatic reticulum, 29
Endothelial damage, 35
Enzyme induction, 28-33
Enzyme inhibition, 30, 31
Epinephrine, 35
Erythromycin, 39
Estrogens, 32, 34, 37, 50
Ethanol, 29, 42
Ethacrinic acid, 34
Ethylene glycol, 50
Excretion, 30, 40, 41
Experimental pathology, 22
Extracellular fluid, 40

False positive results, 16

Fatty acids, 35
Folic acid, 64

Ganglionic blockers, 43
Gastric ulcers, 30
Genetic differences, 32, 34
Glucuronyltransferase, 34
Glycine, 50
Glycolate, 50
Glyoxylate, 50
Goitrogens, 47, 48
GRAS substances, 57
Gray syndrome, 40
Guidelines for safety testing,
  4-9, 14-17
Gunn strain rats, 34

Heinz-Ehrlich bodies, 63
Hemolytic anemia, 54, 55, 63
Heparin, 35
Hepatotoxicity, 30, 40, 42, 64
Hexachlorocyclohexene, 29
Hexachlorophene, 56-59
Hexobarbital narcosis, 29
Hycanthone, 16
Hydralazine, 36
Hypalbuminemia, 34
Hypercoagulability, 35
Hyperoxaluria, 50-52
Hyperthermia, 44
Hypervitaminosis, 60
Hypoprothrombinemia, 30, 31, 63

Infants, 39-42
Inflammatory response, 32
Innocent bystander mechanism, 54
Intracellular fluid, 40
In vitro investigations, 21
Isoniazid, 16, 36, 37, 51, 64
Isoproterenol, 43, 44

Kernicterus, 34
Kideny stones, 50-52

Laughing gas, 29
LD$_{50}$, 23-27, 39-41, 44
Lens opacities, 41, 43
Lincomycin, 39
Lipid solubility, 33
Liver necrosis, 30, 42
Lysosomes, 62

Mefenamic acid, 34
Menadione, 63
Meprobamate, 42
Methemoglobinemia, 63
Methotrexate, 33, 34
3-Methylcholanthrene, 29
α-Methyldopa, 54
Metrazol, 36
Microsomal enzymes, 29-33, 40
Mitochondria, 48-62
Monoamine oxidase inhibitors, 43
  44
Monocrotaline, 40
Monosodium glutamate, 42
Morphine, 41
Moving averages, 26, 27
Mutagenicity, 12-15
Myocardial damage, 43
Myocarditis, acute, interstitial,
  52-53

Nalidixic acid, 34, 41
Neoarsphenamine, 53
Nephrocalcinosis, 62
Nephrolithiasis, 50-52
Nephrotoxicity, 42, 50, 64
Neuroleptics, 43
Neuropathy, 36, 58, 64, 67-71
Neurotoxicity, 36, 42, 57, 64, 67-
  71
Newborn, 39-42
Nicotinic acid, 64
p-Nitrobenzoic acid, 40
Non-hemolytic, unconjugated hyper-
  bilirubinemia, 34
Number of animals, 17-18

Old age, 42, 43
Optical neuritis, 36
Oral contraceptives, 14, 34, 37
Oraganophosphorus insecticides, 30
Orthostatic hypotension, 43
Oxalic acid, 36, 49-52
Oxaluria, 49-52

Pantothenic acid, 64
Penicillamine, 36, 37
Penicillin, 39, 53
Pentobarbital, 41
Pharmaceutical formulation, 20
Pharmacokinetics, 20, 40, 42
Phenacetin, 54
Phenobarbital, 30, 32, 41
Phenothiazines, 44
Phenuridone, 53

Phenylbutazone, 29-32, 34
Physical information, 20
Pitressin, 43
Platelet aggregation, 35
Polycyclic hydrocarbons, 29
Polyphasic dose-effect curve, 25
Preclinical toxicity studies, 8, 9
Pregnancy, 34
Procaine, 36, 44
Propranolol, 43
Protein binding, 33-35, 44, 55
Pulmonary hypertension, 35, 40
Pyridoxal phosphate, 36, 37, 51
Pyridoxic acid, 36

Quinidine, 54
Quinine, 54

Range finding procedure, 26
Reserpine, 44
Retinoic acid, 61
RNA polymerase, 29

Salicylates, 34, 44
Sedormid^R, 54
Semicarbazide, 36
Seizure, 36
Serum albumin, 33-35
Sex differences, 31, 50
Simplified toxicity tests, 26, 27
Skin reactions, 52, 53
SMON, 67-71
Species differences, 29, 31, 33, 40
Spongiform encephalopathy, 57, 58
SQ 18,506, 16
Steroid metabolism 32
Stibophen, 54
Streptomycin, 39
Subacute myelo-optico-neuropathy, 67-71
Subacute toxicity studies, 8, 11, 12
Sulfadimethoxine, 33
Sulfanilamide, 33
Sulfonamides, 33, 34, 47, 53
Sympathomimetic amines, 44

Temperature, 43-45
Teratogenicity, 12-14, 61
Testosterone, 50

Tetracycline, 39
Theophylline, 35
2-Thiobarbituric acid, 47
Thiocyanates, 47
Thiosemicarbazides, 36, 47
Thiouracil, 47, 48
Thrombogenic effects, 19, 35
Thrombosis, 35
Thyroid stimulating hormone, 47
Thyroid stimulation, 46-48
Time of death, 25
Tocopherol acetate, 63
Tolbutamide, 29, 30, 34
Toxicological check list, 19-22
Toxicity rating, 24
Triamcinolone, 25
Trichloroacetic acid, 34

U 11,634, 47
Up-and-down method, 26
Uremia, 35

Vaccine, 53
Vitamin A, 61, 62
Vitamin B$_1$, 64
Vitamin B$_2$, 64
Vitamin B$_6$, 36, 37, 50-52, 60, 63 64
Vitamin B$_{12}$, 64
Vitamin C, 29, 51, 52, 64
Vitamin D, 50, 62, 63
Vitamin E, 63
Vitamin K, 63

Warfarin, 34

Xanthurenic acid excretion, 36, 37

Zoxazolamine paralysis, 29